TERESA FERREIRO VILARIÑO

I HAVE BREAST CANCER

What Now?

I Have Breast Cancer – What Now?

Teresa Ferreiro Vilariño

Translation: Mark Lodge
Illustrations: Josep Maria Casas Tuset
Design: María Benavides
Cover design: Enrique Iborra

ISBN: 978-84-616-7129-8

This book is designed to provide information and motivation to our readers.
It is sold with the understanding that the author is not engaged to render
any type of psychological, legal, or any other kind of professional advice. Its
content is the sole expression and opinion of its author. The author shall not
be liable for any physical, psychological, emotional, financial, or commercial
damages, including, but not limited to, special, incidental, consequential
or other damages. You are responsible for your own choices, actions, and results.

"I proclaimed then… that the brain of man was God's drug-store and had in it all liquids, drugs, lubricating oils, opiates, acids, and anti-acids, and every quality of drugs that the wisdom of God thought necessary for human happiness and health."

ANDREW TAYLOR STILL,
Father of the osteopathy

"Your time is limited, so don't waste it living someone else's life. Don't be trapped by dogma — which is living with the results of other people's thinking. Don't let the noise of others' opinions drown out your own inner voice. And most important, have the courage to follow your heart and intuition."

STEVE JOBS,
Apple CEO and co-funder
Stanford University commencement speech, 2005

Contents

Acknowledgments

A friendly word from some close friends gave me the impetus I needed to turn my experience and my notes into a book. My sincere thanks, dear Klamburg. You too, Fina, for having conveyed so much without even trying. Dora, Ascen, Julia, Alicia, Cocó, Ceres, Ceci, thanks for reading, for offering guidance and for sharing what you know with me.

My editors of the Spanish edition, Anna and Joana deserve a special acknowledgement for having opened their door to me and for receiving me with such affection: for their energy, their time and their enthusiasm. And Juli, thanks for believing in me.

Thanks to my mother for giving me, without my asking, the space I needed. To my family, to my two families, and to Mari Carmen. To all of them for their patience, and for respecting my way of doing things.

Lastly, infinite gratitude to everyone who was there for me during that time you have enriched my experience. To give names would imply excluding so many ...

Josep (Joss), thanks, thanks, thanks!!!

Note from the author

What you will read below describes a personal experience and a way of thinking and of positioning oneself towards illness and towards life. Mine.

In August 2009, I was diagnosed with a breast tumour. I was thirty-six years old. Following a preterm birth during the sixth month of pregnancy that led to the loss of my baby, I was trying to get pregnant once again. On top of that, I wanted to turn my professional career around and had found a job in an excellent business school that made me very happy.

I considered the treatment as another project. I have always approached life this way. I suppose I know no other. And when I discovered I had a tumour, I focused my energies on understanding what was happening to me, what the implications were, how long each stage would last, and what I could do to make it bearable. I refused to accept the doctors' versions, their sententious way of speaking, as they were neither consistent with my values nor with my way of understanding.

The doctors treated my body as if they were individual parts. I understand it as a whole. They asked me nothing, when we hold so many of the answers inside ourselves. They spoke of statistics and of numbers, not of people. And they bandied about categorical assertions, for them irrefutable, of which I was not a participant. I refused to believe them then and I don't believe them now. I looked for other options, tried them, and above all, stayed true to myself, in spite of the doctors' criteria.

When I finished the treatment, in late July of 2010, I gave over all my energy to getting my former life back on track, exactly as I had left it. I continued to set recovery objectives, and each new achievement, each small step, gave me renewed joy.

In September of that same year, I noticed that my right arm was swelling up. It was an effect of the surgery. I had developed lymphedema, and that really was not in my plans. It marked the moment of my emotional downfall, for want of a better name. I had no strength to keep up that positive spirit, for I realized that things would never be the same again. It was a blow. But without it, these notes would not have seen the light of day, because lymphedema heralded a period of reflection that helped me understand. This book brings together that experience, combined with practical information that I found helpful.

It is certainly not my intention to provide advice or magic formulas to solve anyone's problems. I firmly believe that the secret of healing lies primarily in the desire to heal, but that does not mean I'm encouraging people to stop or interrupt treatment. Even having done this myself. Because in doing so, once the positive and negative repercussions and consequences have been assessed, my decision was taken consciously. I want to be consistent, so I accept that henceforth whatever may happen is the result of my choice.

The real message I wish to share is to remember that we have a right to know, to make decisions if we want to. We have a choice. No doctor or family member can compel us to do something we don't want to do. It is essential to look inwards, rather than cast all our hopes and responsibility of healing outwards, to others. Yes, I encourage you to be true to yourselves and to do what you believe appropriate at the time, according to your own criterion.

This book is full of hope and looks fearlessly at illness, with transparency, but without trivializing it. It is written in the feminine for obvious reasons, although it's also addressed to men. The readers I have in my mind are women who have had a tumour detected in their breast, because we have shared a similar experience. I think this compendium of 'tools for approaching and engaging' a breast tumour will most benefit them. If anyone else – close to the experience or not – can benefit from all that I've learned, the gift I have received for having written this book will be a little greater.

Anything can happen and may continue to happen in two, five or ten years. For just as a day starts life, so a day will end it. Knowing and remembering this can help us enjoy a little more, and put in its place what really matters without feeling guilty, and without fear, but with confidence, and at peace.

Foreword

I have had the privilege of knowing Teresa for more than ten years, since she attended an executive program at IMD, where I am the LEGO Professor of Supply Chain. From that moment we became friends. Finally, a couple of years ago, I was lucky enough to convince her to lead the team of an IMD research centre that I direct.

Given my profession, I know little about breast cancer, but I'm constantly dealing with top leaders of big multinationals. Teresa's book is about her journey through breast cancer and also about guiding oneself through a period of crisis and growing personally through that journey. A challenge very similar to what top executives encounter in their professional life.

This is the story of Teresa suddenly being confronted with a world unknown to her, that of cancer specialists, tests, diagnoses and more tests, and the need to make very quick decisions that would have a huge impact on her life. She chose not to be a passenger on a journey that is usually guided by doctors' advice. She decided to take the lead in a situation of ambiguity, uncertainty and anxiety.

She embarked on an amazing task of gathering information, understanding the issues and, crucially, having a critical reading of it all. She also endeavoured to learn about non-traditional views and understand their value in her situation. She does a fantastic job of providing the accepted scientific theories in an understandable way, highlighting the limits of current scientific knowledge and offering a very balanced perspective of non-traditional views that might be very useful for this journey.

It is a masterpiece of how to form one's own judgement about a very important set of decisions for your life and how to deal with the emotions and the impact on it. The book doesn't show an idealistic view of a hero standing strong against adversity, but that of a person going through ups and downs and looking for a way forward.

The parallel with executives or people making decisions when existing knowledge is limited and under the need to redefine objectives is striking. At business schools we teach about making decisions under uncertainty and ambiguity, this book is an ultimate example about it.

I must also add that in her book Teresa explains how she dealt with the external world when undergoing that journey. In particular, she explains how reserved she was and how little she allowed the external world to know about her concerns and remain a business professional. By reading the book it is possible to wonder up to which point the writing is biased. I was with Teresa for much of her journey and I must say that I only discovered what she went through when I read the book. She was very professional and didn't allow her concerns to affect her interactions with friends and business colleagues. Thus, her story is, from my point of view, a very true one that reflects the reality of what she did.

While reading the book and during discussions with executives in which Teresa explained her story, it became evident that many managers found her account a very inspiring one from a leadership point of view. They found it very relevant to their experiences. They considered that it is a story from which they and their colleagues in companies can learn. After reading, witnessing and helping executives to improve their leadership for many years, I believe that stories like this one are the most impactful way of learning.

A final note from the point of view of somebody with a PhD and, therefore, conscious about the constraints of the scientific method. We know that science advances in what is called paradigm shifts, big changes that challenge previously known science. Albert Einstein famous quote is that "if at first, the idea is not absurd, then there is no hope for it". Thus, the wise reader will not discard the theories that the book presents about alternative approaches, even though they are not the mainstream ones. These theories might be proven right by the scientific method in the future. This is the way science advances and Teresa does a great job providing a very balanced view of different theories.

This book is a fascinating story about a person, Teresa, guiding herself through a previously unknown world, finding the resources, the courage and the intellectual capacity to deal with an uncertain and anxious world. It is an inspiring journey that should help the reader to reflect on his or her own life journey.

CARLOS CORDÓN
LEGO professor of Supply Chain Management at IMD

Introduction

The scene may change, but not the essence:

> One day, in the shower, you feel a lump. Of course, it's nothing... You go to the doctor, you are referred to another, you undergo a biopsy... You test positive! Or...

> They phone you. You had a mammogram a few days back. They want you to come in because the results are unclear... You go back, they examine you, a biopsy is taken and... positive! Or...

> You visit the gynecologist for any other complaint, such as ovarian pain. She carries out a complete examination and discovers a lump in your breast. Referred to another specialist, you undergo a biopsy and... positive.

At some point in your life you may find yourself in this position, as one in eight women do, according to the National Cancer Institute (NCI).[1]

And suddenly, the abyss, the haste, the important decisions without having enough information. Even the possibility of death! You are spoken to in terms that were foreign to you until now, of urgent treatments, of surgery and operating theatres. You are spoken to about

---

1. Source: National Cancer Institute: www.cancer.gov/cancertopics/factsheet/detection/probability-breast-cancer

chemotherapy, about radiotherapy, about hormones, about tests and further tests... And you are not quite sure what to hold on to or what to do. There's no time to think. The system is stronger, and you are only given two alternatives: accept the rules and play their game or leave and allow yourself to be racked by the cancer invading your body without treatment. The decision is yours, they say, and you must make it now. Obviously, put in these terms, few women are capable of analyzing the situation and deciding consciously how they want to treat their illness before getting sucked into the vortex. Most of us join the game without assessing it enough, and once inside, or upon completing the process, we wonder if we might not have preferred to do it differently, to have had more information, more time, more resources...

This is how I experienced it, how I felt, and this is the reason I chose to write this book. Because having undergone chemotherapy, surgery, radiotherapy and countless other alternative and complementary treatments, I believe at the time I was lacking answers that I have had to learn to find. It was a year in which I tried a lot, read, made inquiries, listened, learned and understood.

This is why I wish to share my experience, bringing together in a single book the aspects that for me were fundamental to the process you go through when you have been diagnosed with a tumour.

There are no illnesses, but only ill people. And there are no statistics, only human beings. But I will address all this below. Without advice or magic formulas. Because ultimately the most important thing will be the outcome after you close this chapter of your life and start a new one. And the decisions you will have made up until then will have been the right ones, because you did what you believed was appropriate at that juncture.

Chapter One

THE DIAGNOSIS

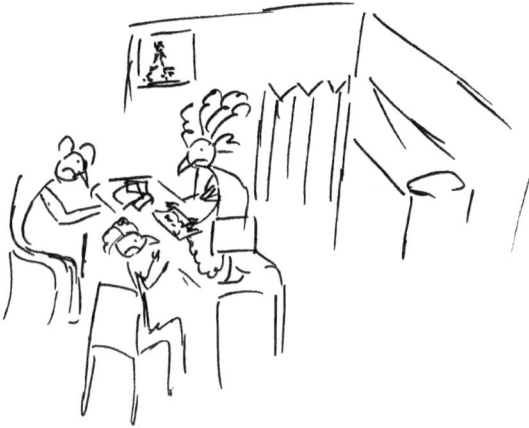

Mine

I had the biopsy in mid-summer, and the doctor in charge told us to do something to take our minds off it over the ten days it would take to find out the results. The doctor didn't want to get ahead of himself, taking a cautious yet realistic stance. So we headed straight from the health clinic to a travel agent, and a few days later we were on the beach.

On our return, we went to see the doctor who henceforth would handle our case (and I say 'our' because while the lump was in my breast, and I was the one who underwent the chemo, my partner was always with me, sometimes going through more difficult moments than I was).

The breast pathology consultant who gave us the results, and who would be our referring doctor, was very straightforward. The biopsy was positive, and we would have to begin treatment as soon as possible. At that time, she preferred not say much else until the results of the other tests came in, but it seemed that chemotherapy was unavoidable.

I was young, I had my life ahead of me, and so, although my tumour was not very aggressive, nor had it spread much, we would attack it with every weapon at our disposal. Put bluntly, they decided to use sledgehammers to crack nuts to be on the safe side.

Leaving the doctor's surgery I felt dizzy, my stomach churning up inside. Joss and I embraced and we soothed each other with cuddling and kisses. No matter how much one prepares for this kind of news, you are never entirely ready. You always hold out the hope that it's a mistake and that the situation will be nicer and more positive than you imagine it will be.

The days went by. I got in touch with a number of different people, learning, listening. It was a time of turmoil and information overload: as you open up a new source of information until then unknown to you, a simple search leaves you overwhelmed with terms. You want to become an expert in the subject matter overnight, to understand it in order to asses it, and at times you get lost and confused because there are so many different opinions, so many contradictions and ways of tackling the same issue that you end up not knowing what is the best for you, which one to choose.

In my case, I doubted everything. The idea of chemotherapy left me cold. I was feeling so well! Barely a year had passed since I'd lost the child we were expecting during my sixth month of pregnancy. It was a tough pregnancy, with constant morning sickness, marked mood swings and a strong feeling of inhabiting a body that wasn't mine, of not being me. Those months put a strain on our relationship. On account of the nausea, I could do almost nothing, I couldn't go for a stroll, drive, go to the cinema, I felt dreadful. I was constantly vomiting, two or three times in the morning, and I felt guilty for it.

Pregnancy was supposed to be a happy experience, yet we were living it like an ordeal. The pregnancy was planned, we wanted to be parents, but nothing transpired as we had imagined it would.

September 8th 2008 unleashed a chain of events that brought my pregnancy to an end. I was feeling bad, with some discomfort. I called the gynecologist to explain my symptoms. She wasn't concerned so we decided to spend the weekend in the mountains. On the evening of September the 8th I was bleeding slightly and felt some cramps, so we went to an accident and emergency room in the early hours. I was sent home with a paracetamol and a medical report suggesting "risk of miscarriage", and I was instructed to rest. We did not read the report until several days later. There was no time. The following morning I was still bleeding and had more intense pains. We took the car, returned to Barcelona, and went directly to the accident and emergency department of the hospital. I had gone into labour. I had dilated more than 6 cm. The doctors told me that it would be very difficult to stop the birth once the contractions started (it seems they were not cramps). Indeed, my body expelled the baby, which at 22 weeks and a day, was too tiny to confront the world on its own. The event had been brought on by an infection in the placenta, as I was to find out three months later.

It was a traumatic moment in my life. I still recall those months of pregnancy with revulsion because of the physical implications involved. If to this we add that I had imagined a natural birth, with my partner at my side holding my hand throughout the process, warm lighting in the room and no medical intervention, without operating theatres, or nurses, or epidurals, you will understand that the reality was no cup of tea. I spent the dilation phase in a cubicle in the emergency room, connected to an intravenous drip that was meant to stop the contractions. When it was inevitable, I was taken to the delivery room. Joss had to wait outside. I was ill prepared, I hadn't even taken the course on how to breathe during childbirth. My body wanted to expel the baby and the rest of me wanted it to stay inside. I was being told to push, but how, and why?

They took away Eloi at birth. I scarcely remember anything. Later they showed him to us. He was tiny and beautiful. He seemed at peace. He had gradually faded away, but hadn't suffered. Seeing him reassured us. He had not suffered. He simply left.

From that month of September until the following summer, Joss and I put all our effort into getting our life back on track. Doing our utmost to overcome the trauma. We did not wish the experience to have a negative impact on us. Clearly, it marked us, but my big obsession was not to let what had happened us create any distance or silence between us. To this end, we addressed the issue openly, we spoke about it frequently and we decided to try pregnancy again after some time. In fact, we had been trying for a few months before they detected my tumour.

Although some doctors insist that there is no connection between the loss of a baby and the emergence of a tumour, I find it hard to swallow. How can two such important events that happen to a person in so short a space of time be unrelated? Moreover, both being directly linked to fertility and femininity. Both so sensitive to hormones. Both so extreme, and so instrumental to life.

After that month of September 2008 in which I went into labour, I focused on my physical and psychological recovery. I wanted to get pregnant again, I wanted to be strong, prepared, and I also wanted to recover the figure I had before. Because, if you have your baby as a final reward, the kilos and flab from pregnancy are more bearable than the ones you carry as the sole memento upon returning from the hospital.

I was exercising several times a week, I watched what I ate even more than before, and I tried to live and enjoy daily life with zest. I was fit, and ready to take on the world once again. I had even found a new job that motivated me and opened up doors to my professional future.

It was in this context that the tumour was found.

Tumour types and phases

Obviously, the first thing I did when I had a moment was to search the Internet for everything I could find about breast tumours. Conventional health professionals advise you not to do this, I imagine because they can't control the information you are accessing. It's true that Internet abounds with nonsense, and that what you read is not necessarily rigorous or even true. But it's also true that we can find reliable sources of information that we can collate by searching different websites and so ensure that what we read is rigorous.

The Internet is a good source of information if we know how to use it and are able to relativize it (a forum discussion is not as reliable as a newspaper article or a paper published in a scientific journal). I encourage you to clear up any doubts if that reassures you, and even to describe your experience on the Web if sharing it helps you. Again, we are what's important, to feel good and seek out environments that give us strength and support.

Described below are the different types and phases of breast tumours, which are defined by four types of parameters:[2]

1. Location of the tumour
2. Biology of the tumour cell
3. The TNM staging system: size, lymph nodes affected and metastasis
4. Histologic tumour grades

---

2. Sources: the American Cancer Society, WebMD, National Cancer Institute and the AECC (Spanish Association Against Cancer).

Types of breast tumours

Based on their location

Anatomically, breast cancer originates in the terminal ductal lobular unit of the mammary gland.

When the malignization process forms in the ducts, ductal carcinoma originates. When it forms in the lobules the result is lobular carcinoma.

The breast is a gland. The tumour arising in the cells and structures of this gland is called breast cancer, thus breast cancer is an adenocarcinoma.

1. *Ductal Carcinoma in situ*
   This is the name given to malignant cell proliferation that occurs inside the milk duct, without breaking growing through its wall (basement membrane), that is, without invading or infiltrating the tissue (stroma) surrounding it. It is called:

   a. *Ductal carcinoma in situ or intraductal carcinoma*
      If the malignancy is in a duct.

   b. *Lobular carcinoma in situ*
      If it is within a lobule.

   The incidence of both types of tumours has increased in recent years. Noteworthy is the frequency with which these forms of highly localized breast cancers are multifocal (several lesions in the same breast) and bilateral (cancer occurring in both breasts). It is not known what percentage of these highly localized tumour types become invasive tumours. The time period over which this happens may be as long as between 6 and 10 years.

2. Invasive (infiltrating) ductal carcinoma

This is the name given to malignant cell proliferation that spreads through the wall of the duct or the lobule, and invades the surrounding tissue. This is the most common type of tumour, accounting for 9 out of 10 breast cancers. There are two main types of invasive breast cancer:

a. **Ductal carcinoma:** it starts in the cells lining the milk ducts (through which milk flows to the nipple). This is the most common type, accounting for 8 out of 10 breast cancers.

b. **Lobular carcinoma:** it originates in the breast lobules, where the milk is produced. It has a far lower incidence of 1 in 10 cases.

c. **Inflammatory breast carcinoma:** a rare but more malignant histological type. The tumour cells infiltrate the lymph vessels and the skin. The breast becomes red all over and feels warm, as if it were inflamed, hence its name. It has a low incidence, accounting for some 1 to 3% of all breast cancers.

d. **Other less common types of breast cancer are:**
- *Medullary*
- *Colloid*
- *Tubular*

3. Paget's disease

Paget's disease of the breast is a condition affecting the skin of the nipple or of the areola, associated or not to an underlying intraductal (*in situ*) or invasive carcinoma.

Today breast cancer is classified according to the biology of the tumour cell. Whether or not it is hormone/endocrine receptor positive, and whether or not the tumour contains the HER2 protein, it will be defined as one of the following types of breast cancer:

1. **Hormone receptor-positive**
   These tumours grow in response to estrogen and progesterone hormones, also known as hormone-dependent tumours. They account for 66% of all breast cancers and are most commonly found in postmenopausal women.

2. **HER2-positive breast cancer**
   The protein HER2 is overexpressed in tumour cells and they do not have hormone (estrogen or progesterone) receptors.

3. **Triple-negative breast cancer**
   Tumour cells lack estrogen or progesterone receptors and do not overexpress the protein HER2. This is a far less common type of cancer, accounting for some 15% of all breast cancers.

4. **Triple-positive breast cancer**
   Tumour cells are responsive to hormones (estrogen or progesterone), but also overexpress the protein HER2. It accounts for some 12% of all breast cancers.

The TNM staging system

The American Joint Committee on Cancer (AJCC) TNM system is most commonly used to describe the stages of breast cancer. The letters refer to three aspects of the cancer:

➤ T

Refers to the size of the tumour or to its spread. The accompanying numbers, from 0 to 4, describe this size (T1 if it is less than or equal to 2 cm, T2 if it is between 2 and 5 cm, T3 if it is bigger than 5 cm) and if it has invaded the surrounding skin or the chest wall under the breast, T4.

➤ N

Indicates whether it has affected the lymph nodes. It is numbered from 0 (which indicates no infiltration of the lymph nodes) to 3 (N1 if 1 to 3 lymph nodes are affected, N2 if 4 to 9 lymph nodes are affected, and N3 if the number is more than or equal to 10, even if the affected lymph nodes are far from the breast).

➤ M

Refers to whether or not other organs are affected. 0 indicates no metastasis, or 1, metastasis.

Clinical stages

According to the *T, N and M* categories, breast cancers are grouped into the following *stages*:

➤ *Stage 0:*

These are pre-malignant lesions, also called carcinoma *in situ*. The tumour cells are located exclusively within the wall of the lobules or the milk ducts.

➤ *Stage I (TI, N0, M0):*
The tumour is less than 2 cm in size. It has not spread to the lymph nodes nor is there distant metastasis.

➤ *Stage II:*
The tumour measures between 2 and 5 cm, and has or has not spread to axillary lymph nodes. It is subdivided into stage IIA (T0, N1, M0 or T1, N1, M0 or T2 N0, M0) and stage IIB (T2, N1, M0 or T3, N0, M0).

➤ *Stage III:*
The tumour affects axillary lymph nodes or skin and chest wall (muscles or ribs). It is subdivided in stage IIIA (T0-2, N2, M0 or T3, N1-2, M0), stage IIIB (T4, N0-2, M0) and stage IIIC (T0-4, N3, M0).

➤ *Stage IV:*
The cancer has spread, affecting other organs such as bone or the liver (any T, any N, M1).

This classification in stages is closely linked with disease prognosis and survival. The five-year survival rate is 100% in stage I and about 20% in stage IV.

Histological tumour grading

The characteristics of malignant cells enable additional classification. The cells that form breast cancers are described according to tumour grade. The grade depends upon the similarity of tumour cells to normal breast cells, suggesting how fast the cancer may grow:

➤ *Grade 1 (well-differentiated):*
The cells look much like normal cells and these tumours grow slowly.

➤ *Grade 2 (moderately-differentiated):*
They bear some resemblance to the original cells and grow faster than grade 1 cells.

➤ *Grade 3 (poorly-differentiated):*
They do not resemble the cells they originated from and grow rapidly. These are the ones that spread most often.

The set of these parameters define the type of tumour and, therefore, the treatment to be performed. One or another protocol is applied depending on the type of tumour.

My tumour was entirely hormone-dependent and HER2 negative; according to the TNM system it was T3 N0 M0. In other words, it was found at stage IIB, (so it measured more than 5 cm to 5.5 cm, to be precise), no lymph nodes were affected and there was no metastasis. Furthermore, it was a slow-growth tumour.

Chapter Two

WHY DO I HAVE A LUMP IN MY BREAST?

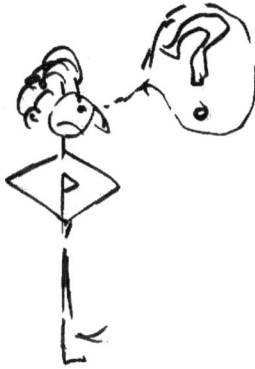

What is it?

This is one of the first questions we ask ourselves, and one of the first to be left unanswered. In a society where ever more women are being diagnosed with breast cancer at a younger age, why do the experts lack an answer to such a simple question?

From Western medicine

Traditional medicine, being a science, has been characterized by its ability to conduct studies and analyse different variables based on research with focus groups, which are sets of people with a characteristic (or disease) in common who undergo the same treatment.

The results obtained lead to conclusions, which are often reflected in statistics or recommendations. For example, "women who have a child before the age of thirty-five years have a lower risk of developing breast cancer."

This type of medicine primarily focuses on tackling the problem, and on this point differs from other types of medicine because Western medicine often qualifies as an illness what other streams of thought consider to be a symptom, i.e., our body telling us that something is wrong.

Western medicine provides fast and accurate solutions. It is extremely effective in solving acute problems (controlling hemorrhages, open heart surgery), and has made great advances and in many directions thanks to the large number of different specialists who have focused on understanding a specific organ of our body.

From their knowledge, many doctors have developed new lines of knowledge that seek solutions to the problem from inside rather than outside the body.

A good example of this way of practising medicine is Andrew Taylor Still, the father of osteopathy. Osteopathy bases health on the proper functioning of our body from a mechanical point of view, in which the structure of bones, muscles and nerves are able to operate freely, without obstacles. Using his body manipulation therapy Still was able to restore health to sick people. He once said that "The brain of man was God's drug-store and had in it all liquids, drugs, lubricating oils, opiates, acids, and anti-acids, and every quality of drugs that the wisdom of God thought necessary for human happiness and health".[3] Therefore, if the brain is the world's most comprehensive pharmacy, we just have to give our body a chance and make it as easy as possible for it to act.

There are many more examples of medical researchers who have broken new ground in science, such as Dr Budwig, who we shall discuss in the chapter on nutrition.

---

3. STILL, A.T. (1981), *Autobiography of A. T. Still*. Indianapolis: American Academy of Osteopathy.

We know that a tumour is a mass of cells grouped together which, due to a mutation our body has failed to control, begin to reproduce rapidly and abnormally. These cells are destructive and can spread to the rest of the body if they are not detected and treated early, when they are still located in the form of lump in a specific part of our body. But despite its efforts, Western medicine has not been able to find a satisfactory answer to the question:

Why do cells mutate?

Given that Western medicine has not found a satisfactory answer to date, I wanted to find one from other sources and other types of medicine.

Dr Hamer's theory

Ryke Geerd Hamer was born in Mettmann (Düsseldorf, Germany) in 1935. He studied medicine, specialized in internal medicine, and worked for two years together with his wife, an oncologist, with cancer patients.

In 1978, he had a life-changing experience. His son died of cancer. Soon after, Hamer himself developed testicular cancer, and his wife, breast cancer. It was then when he pondered the relationship between the two diseases and began to conduct research. He worked on the hypothesis that a psychological shock can trigger different types of cancer. They are what he termed 'biological conflicts.'

First, he began to ask patients about their lives. Hamer tried to find out if they had suffered any trauma in the years prior to the onset of their cancer. In all the cases he found that the answer was yes. It's worth bearing in mind that oncologists never pose this question to their patients.

The research led him to perform brain scans on a large number of patients, thanks to which he discovered that different types of cancer can be diagnosed from CT brain scans, in which they are reflected. Dr Hamer found that the same disease always correlates with the same place in the brain. Thus, women who have had a breast tumour will have a common lesion on their brain scan.

Dr Hamer went even further in his discoveries. By studying his patients, he realized that similar emotional traumas generate the same disorder in different patients. In the case of breast cancer, Hamer speaks of a sense of abandonment, traumatic loss. However, he also explains that it is not always easy to establish the trauma that triggers the disease. In some people, the disease takes years to develop for various emotional reasons (low self-esteem, resentment, anger, feelings of injustice).

For Germanic New Medicine, a school that arose from Hamer's research and that draws together and supports all its principles, that which is defined as a disease by standard medical terms, is actually a healing process that our body uses to overcome certain situations. Therefore, without medical intervention, but rather conscious and active work by the patient to overcome and heal his or her emotional trauma, in addition to other therapeutic measures defined by the patient and agreed upon by most alternative therapies to Western medicine (food, attitude, etc.), one can neutralize and eliminate the tumour.

In conclusion of his work, Hamer formulated the *Five Biological Laws*, which is based on studying the human being as a whole. Our body and our cells are not independent from our mind and our feelings. So, emotions or traumatic experiences can create organic imbalances that become illnesses.

1st law:

Diseases originate from an acute shock event that, depending on the feeling generated by the patient's subjective experience, is reflected in a location in the brain and in the relevant organ.

This process occurs simultaneously in the psyche, the brain and the organ itself.

2nd law:

Intensifies into the phases of the illness.

3rd law:

Explains the correlation between the psyche, the brain and the organs.

4th law:

Describes the biological purpose of the fungi and microorganisms that inhabit our body.

5th law:

Disease has a biological meaning and a purpose, which is to resolve a conflict.

Dr Hamer is a controversial figure. He himself was aware of the difficulties that could – and in fact, did – arise around his theory. Indeed, Germanic New Medicine urges its patients to undergo their treatment discreetly, avoiding lawsuits and disputes with third parties. The patient needs to focus all his or her energy and consciousness inwards and towards personal healing; they cannot afford to squander their energies trying to convince others of the validity of Dr Hamer's theories. The power of their environment is huge, and negative comments do nothing but pose a handicap.

Regardless of the position we defend, Dr Hamer and his proposals are immensely interesting. The way he approaches disease provides food for thought. We are not machines, we are people. If it is currently accepted that stress lowers the body's defences and promotes the spread of infections, why not take it a little further? At the end of the day, cancer also develops following a drop in our immune system defences. In fact, throughout our life, our body produces many malignant cells, but if you are strong and healthy, it is able to identify and neutralize them. Therefore, these cells neither spread nor multiply uncontrollably, since they cease to exist before this can occur.

Part of the doctor's work involved drawing up correlation tables from which deduce the type of disease that can be developed from a type of traumatic event (or vice versa). In the case of breast cancer, this is correlated with experiences of a sudden loss of loved ones, abandonment, maternity-related problems and so forth.

Before learning of Dr Hamer, my intuition already told me that there necessarily had to be a relationship between my pregnancy, preterm birth and the appearance of the tumour. Hamer's theories only served to confirm this.

The point of view of Traditional Chinese Medicine

The origins of Traditional Chinese Medicine (TCM) date back over five thousand years. It is a preventative medicine and its objective is to keep us healthy: prevention more than healing.

Human beings are energy that flows through our body through meridians. Meridians are our 'energy highways.' Of the hundreds of meridians running through our body, twelve of them are considered fundamental. When energy flows properly, our body and our emotions are in balance. We enjoy full health. The problem arises when this balance is upset, generating energy voids and stagnation which result in disease. Therefore, the first concept that sets Western medicine apart from TCM is that disease is a consequence, the end of a process, while for Western medicine disease is the beginning.

TCM does not focus so much on the signs and symptoms of diseases, but rather on the long-term disruptions which are slowly upsetting the balancing of the whole body. That is, in the case of a lump in the breast, the healing process offered by TCM does not begin by removing the tumour. Its disappearance is the final consequence and the final result of a treatment that begins by identifying the cause that is giving rise to the tumour. Clearly it is a disruption in the body.

For some reason, signals sent by our brain are not appropriate because there is an imbalance. And the causes behind this imbalance may be emotional in nature. How we feel can affect our energy. So healing begins by modifying these signals sent by the brain. It is the job of TCM masters to bring about this change and eliminate the stagnation or make our energy flow smoothly. These 'masters' are doctors who use various diagnostic methods, acupuncture needles, and phytotherapy (the science of using plants for therapeutic purposes) to rebalance our energy and restore our health. Their work focuses on the twelve main meridians, as they are the most superficial and accessible from outside the body.

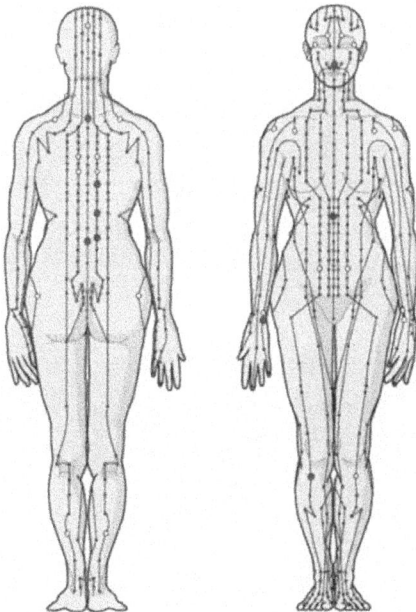

Meridians[4]

_____

4. www.ademedicos.com

In the case of the presence of a tumour, once treatment with TCM has begun, instead of generating malignant cells we begin to generate what is needed to block, inhibit and finally eradicate these cells. Hence the disappearance of the tumour takes place in the last phase of the healing process. First of all, the body needs to understand what is happening in order to regain balance. Having achieved this first goal, it can begin to solve the problem.

From this point of view, once the breast tumour has been treated and overcome there is no place for metastasis, because the body has already found its balance, it has been able to heal and has recovered.

Dr Hamer and TCM doctors are not the only ones to explain the relationship of our body with our mind and our emotions, and treat the individual as a whole. These are only two medical schools of thought, but there are many more (Ayurvedic medicine, to cite another example). In fact, if you look at the ways different cultures approach human health, one realizes that only Western medicine, as practiced today, understands and treats the individual by parts, specializing in organs and systems, rather than treating it as a whole in which all parts are interconnected.

Chapter Three

BEFORE COMMENCING THE TREATMENT

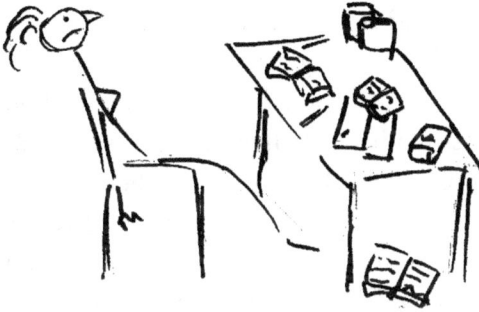

W̲hen you get your biopsy results, thus begins a race against time to save your life, in which every minute, every hour, counts. This is how it was put to me. And I asked myself...

Is this how they want me to feel?

At times like these, one's head begins to reel like a carrousel. Everything feels completely unreal. Just a few days ago you were leading a normal life, but now it seems if you let one more second pass, you are practically signing your own death sentence. In a matter of hours your life has become besieged with words and concepts hitherto unknown to you. They urge you to make hasty decisions, with barely any knowledge. It seems as if they don't want you to have any criteria, your own opinion. The sooner you start the better. Today, tomorrow, in two days' time. They don't seem to realize that one needs a little time to digest what is happening to you and take the plunge consciously. No, **they neither let you speak nor doubt. As if doubting or asking them questions would question the validity of the treatment or cast doubt on their professionalism. And, in truth, this is not what you question. It's your incredulity that is reflected in this doubt, your bewilderment over something you were not expecting.** And you yourself, perhaps thanks to the peace of mind it gives one to recall that moment with hindsight, cannot stop wondering ... Why are they pushing me like this towards fear? Why so much interest in doing things in a rush? According to the Surveillance, Epidemiology and End Results (SEER) Program of the National Cancer Institute, 98% of women who have had a breast tumour without lymph node involvement are still alive after five years[5]. The SEER also estimates that 89.2% of those affected in the United States – without differentiating the extent of the tumour – are still alive after five years. These are amazingly positive statistics. The numbers speak for themselves.

Why all the drama? Why the urgency? They will tell you that it's thanks to this urgency that the statistics are so positive, yet they don't seem to realize that, for the patient, who is not psychologically prepared, a week's reflection before beginning treatment is surely much more valuable than allowing oneself to be directly and blindly sucked into a vortex of urgent processes. Without a modicum of reflection, they introduce a number of additional unnecessary elements of stress and fear that are detrimental to the eventual recovery process. Let's get a sense of proportion.

I'm lost

I don't know what to believe or who to believe in or to listen to. Everyone has an opinion. Everyone knows someone who has been there. And everyone, absolutely everyone, recommends something, an alternative therapy, a doctor, an association...

---

5. Source: http://seer.cancer.gov/statfacts/html/breast.html

Surely this is one the most characteristic feelings common to all at this time. The flood of information leaves you feeling overwhelmed. The news is difficult enough to assimilate in itself. From the moment you learn you have a tumour, in one way or another you have to adapt your life to the new and exceptional situation that implies changes. And changes, as we know, are difficult. If to this we add the heightened sense of ignorance and uncertainty surrounding us, things becomes increasing complicated. Our bodies and minds go into 'alert mode'.

We want to know, and we ask questions. Yet at the same time, faced with the answers, our mind goes blank to protect us – no matter how we have led our life until now, and the decisions we have had to make. Even if we thought we would have a clear position regarding the treatment to follow, in case we were one day faced with this experience, we will probably be surprised by how we feel and think about something we never believed would happen to us.

Who to listen to? What decisions to make?

First of all, I believe it's important to accept the vertigo we feel towards the unknown as part of the process. It is said that among the situations that generate the most stress in a person's life are moving house and changing jobs, for it is in these moments that we dismantle the structures on which we had organized our life. Everyday reality is important, it gives us security. And the environment in which we move in our daily life helps to create ties and references that allow us to feel relaxed. When we are faced with something new, we are immediately put on guard in order to analyze whether it's good or bad, suitable, appropriate … When we move to a new city we will look for the dentist we like, the baker, the mechanic… Because only then will we feel at ease with the knowledge that if the car, for example, has a problem, we know the place where to get it repaired without feeling we've been conned.

The situation is similar when they tell us we have a tumour. And it's hard to come to terms with this, because in all probability you will not have noted any physical change, so, rationally, your head does not see the need to start any treatment. Still, you will have to do it, whatever that is, and surely it will transform your daily life. The foundations and the routine will change drastically and unexpectedly, with the turmoil that this entails.

Therefore, it's essential to accept as something normal the stress due to the new phase that is about to begin. Your entire system will be on guard to experience this situation as well as possible. At times you will get stuck, feel afraid or frustrated and powerless by so many voices around you. When you feel like this, it's important to return to the source: you yourself.

Remember who you are, and what you are like. The most important answers come from within us. Chaos and anxiety may impede us from hearing what our inner self is telling us, knowing what we really want. In these cases, *it is best to listen to your heart.*

And how do we do this?

I believe, deep down, we all know the answers, though it's hard to access them. If you imagine the different choices you have to make, and the options explained to you, some will probably seem easy while others will be tough, imposed somehow by reason, but with background noise, like a high-pitched screech... This is the key to making decisions.

One of my first decisions before starting chemotherapy was to visit a homeopath. I had heard wonderful things about this woman. She had had breast cancer a few years back, and offered some natural treatments that helped to alleviate the side effects of chemotherapy.

Our visit lasted an hour, during which I was extremely sincere, explaining how I had felt up to that point, the projects I had planned for myself in the short term (up to the time of the diagnosis), and how

I wanted to move forward and get on with my life after the treatment. I told her of the tools that were available to me, my own strength to move forward, and the emotional support around me and which nurtured me. She listened to me, and questioned this support. She made a seemingly harmless remark at the time, but that later I realized had left me shaken: "Neither you nor I nor anyone else can do magic. Some things are what they are."

I left her office feeling ill at ease. Something screeched inside me, and I did not know what. I went to the pharmacy to buy the products she had prescribed. I continued feeling apprehensive. Until then I had not doubted myself, or how to address the experience of the tumour.

My steps were self-confident and secure. I was clear I had the resources within me, that my way of going through the process was to challenge what they call cancer and society, and refuse to accept the stigma of the disease. I would not fall into self-pity or victimhood, because I never had done so and also because those feelings shape society's attitude towards cancer, but they were not mine. Cancer was no longer a foreign word or someone else's illness. It was inside me.

And when I paused to listen and feel, my inner voice did not speak the same language as that fearful and alarmist society. My voice spoke of a process, of a possibility to search. My body warned me, and the task that lay before me was to understand what had happened in my life over the years to unleash the cancer. Without guilt, without remorse, and without judgement. We are what we are, and we live as we learn and according to the choices we make. As I see it, my great gift has been to understand why I have lived as I have lived and why I have been as I have been. I have no plan to artificially change that which, according to Hamer, may have triggered the proliferation of malignant cells. It's enough to have understood it and live accordingly, letting go. This is why my conversation with the homeopath made my ears screech so much. She had called into question my beliefs. And in one way or another, to accept her treatment meant choosing between what was outside (this doctor, considered so good and effective) or what is inside (me).

I grasped the situation after several tough days. I chose to stick tight to my beliefs and live accordingly. Henceforth, I told myself: I will base my decisions on what makes me feel good, calm and at peace. That is how I would gauge my actions.

At times like this, when I needed to hear and understand myself, silence, meditation and music were a great help. We all have songs that connect us with the best of ourselves. In my case, it was the songs of Luis Eduardo Aute that took me to that place where I could discover myself with no restraints. His music and philosophy have accompanied me since adolescence, reminding me of the kind of person I want to be. And throughout my experience with the tumour, listening to his albums again helped me to get in touch with my essence and restore my peace of mind.

Obviously, I did not return to the homeopath, nor did I take her medicines. And I think I was right.

Why me?

Again, we can approach this question from several points of view:

Conventional medicine approach

According to the National Cancer Institute,[6] one in eight women will, at some point in their life, find a tumour with carcinogenic characteristics in their breast. These statistics also incorporate environmental factors (exposure to radiation or pollution in the area where you live, your lifestyle) and hereditary factors. Therefore, the likelihood that it will affect you is not so low. A person is more likely to have a breast tumour than to change nationality, for example. The odds of passing a civil service exam or a university or college entrance exam are much higher, and no one makes a big deal in these cases. Therefore,

---

6. Source: National Cancer Institute: www.cancer.gov/cancertopics/factsheet/detection/probability-breast-cancer

according to this line of reasoning we can conclude that it is simply a question of chance.

Integrative or holistic medicine

Our body is the most perfect machine that is known to exist. When we are born it behaves harmoniously. It is programmed to function properly and, if any problems arise, it 'repairs', and even regenerates itself. Always seeking balance and health.

* * *

In the face of an attack, our body, like our mind, reacts. Sometimes it's easy and tangible to perceive the consequences of these reactions, and less so at other times. Dysfunction is evident when the manifestation of these reactions is illness. Something is not working and the human body seeks the means to heal it. We can directly attack the illness itself, or look for the root causes that have led to the dysfunction.

In his book, *Messages from Water*,[7] Masaru Emoto, reveals a surprising world. Like many other researchers, he believes in the memory of water, in its energy and its consciousness. In an attempt to understand better its behaviour, he conducted a comprehensive study in which he analyzed different water samples and then photographed them.

Water molecules, when frozen, group themselves into clusters. The structures forming the molecules differ depending on the characteristics of the water. Spring water, for example, will form beautiful geometric shapes, while polluted water will not. These shapes are the *memory of water*. They transmit a message, their energy. Flowing water, which is oxygenated and is in contact with pristine nature is *living water*. On the other hand, stagnant water, piped and treated for human consumption, is often lacking vital energy. It is called *dead water*. Surprisingly, water does not remain static and isolated from its environment. On the contrary, it is incredibly sensitive to the emotions around it, which it accumulates and embodies. The photographs that

---

7. EMOTO, Masaru. *The Hidden Messages in Water*. Atria Books.

Dr Emoto took of water crystals during his years of research show us how their shapes vary according to what they were exposed to. Dr Emoto exposed different samples of the same distilled water to different stimuli. In some cases, he wrote words on the bottles such as 'Love', 'Thank you', 'I hate you', 'Stupid'.

He exposed other samples to the sound of heavy metal or classical music. Upon analyzing the crystals, Emoto observed that the shape acquired by the water varied. Thus, the crystals of the vial labelled 'Love' were clean, harmonious and perfect. However, those labelled 'I hate you', acquired unattractive and chaotic structures, instead of forming crystals. Therefore, water not only has memory, is also has *consciousness*. It responds to stimuli, and is sensitive to energy vibrations emitted by words (the same word with positive connotations written in different languages formed different crystals, all of them beautiful and consistently arranged), music, and feelings.

A further step in his research led Emoto to discover that water is also able to change its environment. Living water takes on the resonance of charged energy, and transmits life. Dead water is lacking in this vital energy and thus may end up generating illness.

Our body is made up of roughly 70% water. Our thoughts are like words written on a bottle, like music that envelops and modulates us. Our body is not alien to our environment, or our thoughts and feelings. Just as water expresses itself from the stimuli to which it is subjected, so do our cells. Happiness is above all an attitude that does not depend on what is happening in our life, but on how we choose to approach the situations we live through. And each of us has the responsibility and ability to act on our thoughts, our emotions, our desires.

When we choose to be happy our body hurts less, we recover from illnesses faster, because we ourselves induce a healing effect on our system. When we believe in ourselves we find it easier to go further. Illness may be a consequence of approaching life with sadness, anger or bitterness, of the messages we have been sending to ourselves, to our water. Yet we are not here to judge ourselves, but to understand something more, as far as possible, and to act accordingly. Because only when we understand can we begin to change, step by step, the behaviours and attitudes which will help us be happier and lighten our load.

So, we may need to reformulate the question heading these paragraphs. It is not "why me?" but rather "what is this thing that has happened to me trying to tell me, and how I can heal myself?".

Rephrasing the question helps us to see life from a point of view that until now we had not considered. In doing so, we may obtain clues to help us find answers. All scientists agree that stress can cause cancer. Now we can discern a little more clearly the reason why. If every day, for years, we live in a state of anxiety, disappointed by what we do, dissatisfied, in a rush and overwhelmed, what messages are reaching our cells? Illness may be the best warning, because it helps us to stop and reassess our life. It is one more process we have to overcome, from which we will emerge stronger.

Am I going to die?

The big question. The question we all have asked ourselves. Several times, re-reading my notes and drafts, I wondered whether it would be better, less risky, to put aside this paragraph and move on with the book, as if I hadn't thought about this prospect. But I couldn't ignore it because this is precisely where we find the key to the message and to one's own existence.

Society and history have afforded tumours, cysts and other abnormal bodily lumps with enormous power. I don't want to be naïve and nonchalantly suggest that having a tumour is like having a boil. No. But nor do I think to be accurate the message of horror, disease, death and desolation conveyed by the word cancer. It does not match up with reality. At least in the case of the breast tumour I have experienced.

People have died, and die of many things. Not so long ago, any infection, even a toothache, could spell the end. Gradually, thanks to science, to the endless hours researchers have dedicated and the understanding of our own essence as human beings, with the help of thinkers of all types, we have steadily made headway.

I think it's important to highlight the work undertaken by thinkers and experts of our psyche, because their advances are less evident than those of science, but just as real. Therapies, humane treatment and conscious work can cure us of our allergies, phobias, depression. This we know today. It has been demonstrated, and yet, this is not the message one recalls when we are diagnosed with a tumour. We just think that our life has been compromised by something happening to us, something that has taken many people to the grave. And it's important to understand that we can die of a tumour as we can die of many other things. A tumour is not synonymous with death, or misfortune. **Having a tumour doesn't place a curse on you, or turn you into an outcast or a wretch. Having a tumour is just one of the many things that can happen to us in life.** And the best way to overcome the process is to internalize it and accept it as one more stage in your life, a place you've come to – surely for some reason (it's up to each of us to do this internalization work) – and for which you are prepared.

Careful, this doesn't mean that the treatment (whether chemotherapy or anything else) is not necessary. It is essential to act responsibly. But responsibility includes taking charge of the process, because we are the only ones with the right to make decisions concerning our lives, not the doctors. It is important to be informed, to listen to ourselves, learn and make this moment the beginning of a transition to another point in which judgement and the opinions of others will no longer have the importance they once had; there will no longer be so many obligations, and life will become a little lighter, less serious. We will understand that nothing is so transcendent, that our very existence will be a cause for joy without having to look any further.

How do I explain it to people?

Of everything entailed in having a lump in my breast, including the treatment and its side effects, operations, doctors' appointments, visits and so forth, what most upset me was the thought that people would start to feel pity for me.

This is precisely because, as we have seen, the word *tumour* carries tragic connotations; knowing that someone close to you has one can generate feelings of panic in your environment, which is of no help whatsoever.

Even today people utter "Poor thing". And this reaction, whether you like it or not, is overwhelming. Is this why I decided to write this book? Because I got tired of the uphill battle to defuse those feelings with which people identified me?

You most likely feel strong and optimistic about the process you're going through, because you know what you feel, you are living with it from morning to night, knowing you're closer to the end of this stage. Everyone else lives your experience from a distance, often drowned in that sea of sorrow we encountered when talking to doctors, going to hospitals or reading harrowing stories.

Talking about your tumour is your decision, and whatever choice you make will be the right one. However, before you decide, pause to think about the impact of the choice you make.

Confronting the situation head-on
and telling everyone around you that a lump has been discovered in your breast and as a result you will begin treatment is one possibility. If you do, they will ask you questions. They will want to know what treatment you will follow, and they will want to be kept updated. Coming from you, they will consider it reasonable to explain it to others. Soon many more people than you imagine will know. If you are protective of your privacy and don't want to become the subject of conversation, this situation could affect you, because the process you're going through is an intimate and personal experience. Also, knowing that so many people are aware of what's going on in your life may make you feel exposed and vulnerable. Why deny it: Sometimes the misfortunes of others become table talk, and

depending on who's doing the talking it may spark fatalistic connotations, which are so inappropriate.

Sharing it with those close to you,
on the other hand, can be helpful, because by openly expressing it you hear yourself speaking out loud and this will help you to come to terms with it. Also, your friends and family can be a good source of support and affection.

If you say nothing
some people may find you a bit strange, detached and inaccessible. Your reactions may be unexpected or unusual (maybe you don't feel like going to a dinner) and you find yourself giving – and even inventing – excuses to avoid the issue. The advantage here is that people will treat you as before, without deference or compassion. And when they ask how you are, it won't be 'how are you coping' but the same old question.

Your most immediate family
requires another approach. Because it's not so much a question of hiding the situation, in my opinion, as how you convey to them your view of the process, and help them to accompany you with your same energy. We suffer most for our loved ones. We want to protect them from unnecessary anguish and it's not easy to find the best way.

It's best to remember what you already know and latch onto that certainty so you don't get swept away by emotions, and so you can banish in one fell swoop any negative thoughts that may arise. If you talk to your parents, remember you belong to different generations. Surely they have seen friends and family succumb to a tumour, so you might start by explaining how things are now, how far we have advanced. If they see you smile and play it down, they will follow your example, because they will listen to what you want to tell them.

If you have to break the news to your children it's best to speak naturally and be honest. It may be the start of a difficult stage, in which physically you cannot be at your best as usual, but this will not last forever. As quickly as it started, it will soon end. And every day is one day less.

In my case, I did a little of everything. My initial reaction was not to tell anyone. I had no choice but to accept that the people whom I had to see on a daily basis would know. But that was all. I did not want anyone else to know: not friends or acquaintances, let alone strangers! The day I told my parents I asked them not to make it public. They live in a smaller town than mine. They have a close-knit circle of friends. And I know that at times my parents must have needed to share their feelings. But I found it hard to accept that people would know about my most intimate moments. I'm used to controlling what happens in my environment.

To some extent, the professional life I have led up to now explains my reasoning. Working on projects for a multinational company with high demands and limited timeframes has made me what I am. Almost every aspect of my work calls for designing a plan, a strategy, a way to address problems, with a list of actions that must be carried out in a concrete time and a list of people involved in this work, with specific responsibilities. So I approached the tumour and treatment in the same way. As something that had to be accomplished, with times, deadlines, milestones and, obviously, with the best result. From the outset I told myself: I can handle this, and I'll amaze the doctors with my evolution.

Therefore, as a result of my attitude towards my tumour, my mother lived my tumour in her way, as best as she could, as did my father, my siblings, my partner's family and my friends. They virtually excluded me from their conversations with others, if they had them. I was able to avoid comments like "Sandra sends her love," or "Well, you know Carols' daughter also had it". All those things people say with great displays of affection, no doubt, but that weren't going to help me. I tend to say little about what is really important to me in life, because knowing that others know makes me feel vulnerable. The idea that people knew I had a tumour made me feel weak and exposed and I needed to be stronger than ever, to believe that I was in control of what was happening around me. Then nothing could make me fall. Obviously, control is a flight of fancy.

But at least I could plan my day every morning. I chose to confine myself to my small universe, in which I more or less knew what was happening. It was structured around routines like my morning shower, yoga, hospital appointments and alternative treatment appointments, with few surprises. I lived flexibly, depending on my mood and the energy with which I got up that morning, without exposing myself to situations that might be emotionally aggressive. I knew what was really important: my partner, my family, my friends and myself.

It is interesting to see how people react to the same situation. I have two brothers and the way they experienced my condition was completely different. The eldest was more deeply involved: he would call, he took an active interest, providing spiritual support to my mother, listening to her and downplaying the drama of the matter, and he kept informed about each step we took. He was a key figure of support for me because he took charge of mitigating the tough moments that the people close to us might experience. His protection was such that his presence and attitude averted Joss and me from having to deal with difficult conversations.

My other brother, who is a physician, curiously chose to live my process from a distance. He was going through a difficult time, and I imagine that his own situation was hard enough to handle in and of itself. Or maybe he just chose not to get too involved. The truth is that I barely had any contact with him during that year.

In principle I didn't want my friends to tell their friends either. I did not want to be on anyone's lips. And regarding work, the tumour was diagnosed as I was about to start a new project, which I never actually took on, so I did not have to justify myself with explanations. I took an active role in a new professional initiative that kept me occupied and filled those months with enthusiasm and friendship. It was a project with its own times and course. It was an added gift, rich in surprises, affection and warmth.

However, my attitude towards the situation eventually changed and led me to understand that I am not important enough as to be the centre of conversation, and even if I were it would not affect me much. Who was I kidding? No matter how much information I concealed, it was obvious that my life would no longer be the bed of roses I had imagined. I would have preferred nothing to have happened, to not have lived such a harsh experience so young. My experiences are what they are, and they are neither more nor less severe than anyone else's.

We know so little about people. Even a seemingly monotonous or linear life probably has its share of hair-raising experiences. What for us are minor changes can be an abyss for others. It's not what happens to you that is important, but how you perceive it, the importance you attach to it, how you let it unfold and how you let it affect you. Because, again, you have to take your destiny into your own hands.

After all, however much we set our minds to it, however many instructions we give, we have no control over who knows or doesn't know, and who tells or doesn't tell other people what they know. As an example, allow me to explain an experience I had with my sister-in-law, my brother's wife. She is a doctor, and we talk regularly. I kept her up to date on my progress. Respecting my wishes, she kept everything secret until the end. We have been friends since childhood, we went to school together. I have known her siblings for many years. She never told them a thing. During my radiotherapy their little daughter was to be christened, and I took advantage of the occasion to make my 'debut' at the end of whole process. Knowing how I felt, we waited until my hair grew a bit before arranging the celebration.

Of course my extremely short hair immediately drew attention. What's more, I was much thinner. But we could shrug it off as the time of year. Her conduct allowed me to feel comfortable and safe, to avoid having to give explanations and to simply enjoy the christening and the family reunion. I felt really good. But imagine my surprise

– and my sister-in law's – when months later, her father asked after me and went on to say he could no longer pretend he knew nothing, as my uncle had told him everything during the christening! Knowing this now makes me smile.

How to approach it

Confronted with the demoralizing blow of learning you have a tumour, it's best to stop, calm down and reflect. We have already discussed how the system impels you to make hasty decisions. It immerses you in an atmosphere of fear that leaves you blank. You feel it's essential to react in a week, when in fact that tumour takes months to grow, so a little more time, in general, will not change the situation drastically.

We need time for the news to sink in, to assimilate and be able to react to it accordingly. I suppose the immediacy of today (everything is only a click away) has spread to every aspect of life. And we forget that the human being, our mind, needs time to process the information. Listening is often not enough to understand. It's just the first step. Then we begin to make sense of the message in our heads, to digest and assimilate it.

You may need more than a day or two. And it doesn't matter if the doctors already know which procedure to follow from beginning to end, and therefore think they can get ahead of themselves: because what we are embarking on will not be their path, it will be ours. Therefore it is important, indeed essential, that they grant us this time. We should allow ourselves the opportunity to feel lost, confused, scared, hesitant, insecure... All this may happen. And it is precisely during this period when our perspective on the situation will be key to the rest of the process. Because we are searching inwardly for the resources to help us cope with what is to come. Allowing the doctors to decide for us because they are better informed will weaken us. At some point we will doubt whether we have done the right thing or not.

If, on the other hand, we put ourselves first, and from there authorize the doctors' recommendations because we truly believe in them and their knowledge, if we express our confidence in them, their actions will make sense. We will be consistent and accept the stages more easily.

> *We need time to adapt to our new situation. We need to prepare ourselves emotionally, and we need to resolve some practical issues before commencing the process. A day or two will not determine the outcome of treatment, but it can give us the breathing-space we need to assimilate the process with a new attitude. It is essential we give ourselves this time.*

In the time between the diagnosis and starting treatment it seems everything we have discussed thus far is expected of you: knowing what to do, who to tell, accepting what's happening to you, knowing how to react, and so on. This is the time when everyone offers advice without being asked, and tells you that they have friends or relatives who have gone through the same situation, who had this treatment or that. You will be exposed to information overkill.

Your decision as to the approach you take may differ from that of your loved ones, or your partner. It often happens. I know of many cases where, like my own, the patient preferred a less aggressive treatment, while her partner opted for the complete treatment. Such a complicated situation can be further compounded by meaningless remarks from third parties, opining (yet again without your asking them) that in the end it's your life and yours alone and only you can make the decision, not your family. I don't think that's entirely true. In my case, at least, it was essential to maintain a strong bond with my partner, because part of my strength stemmed from our relationship of mutual support and trust.

Each person's circumstances will be very different. The scenario described here reflects one of many that may arise. I understand that there may be people who face the process alone. Their feelings at this point will probably be very different.

At any rate, whether you are alone or if you have a big family, a partner or friends who want to offer their advice, give yourself permission to trust in yourself.

The opinion of others (including mine) may be well-meaning but meaningless, because no one shares your experiences and innermost feelings, and they don't know, therefore, what drives you. Besides, they often don't know how to react, resorting instead to platitudes or clichéd advice without being invited. It's up to us to decide if their advice is sound or simply meaningless.

My life was not mine alone. I was sharing it with a wonderful man who gave me the best and continued doing so without expecting anything in return, and without reproach. He was always there for me. Putting up with my nausea, mood swings, doubts, complaints... My partner and my relationship with him is still today the best gift life has given me.

Did I want to put up more barriers between us than those that arose without looking for them? Was I going to allow outsiders to meddle and give their opinion about an issue that concerned mainly the two of us?

Luckily, I ignored it. When we spoke of chemotherapy, Joss was clear, very clear. He is a scientist and didn't want to leave any stone unturned if it could be avoided. He believed in chemo. And we both wanted to get through this new rough patch.

As I said, I had my doubts. Chemo, I was told, ravages you. Sometimes it stops your period from coming. I wanted to get pregnant. I did not want to have another bad year. Maybe there were other ways... at the end of the day, it was not an aggressive tumour... Besides, my dear Dr Jin, a TCM master who was with me throughout the entire process, and whom I will discuss later, saw no need for chemotherapy. And if Master Jin was of this opinion, so was I.

Despite these doubts, I underwent eight sessions of chemotherapy. I followed the protocol to the letter. After weighing up the pros and cons, I believed it was worth doing because the chemo was important for Joss and Joss was important for me. I preferred to take the path hand-in-hand with Joss and undergo the chemo rather go it alone. Treatment is one more tool, with its benefits and drawbacks. However, relationships are nurtured over a long time, with affection, effort and energy, in which both partners do their part. Finding someone with whom you can be yourself is not easy. Is it worth throwing this priceless gift away for a misconceived loyalty to oneself? I preferred to sustain the strength of our union rather than risk breaking it out of stubbornness. Today I have no regrets. The chemotherapy is over. It had its time, and its consequences, which I gradually overcame. The relationship is still there, stronger than ever.

I know I still have some way to go until my cells return to normal. But it is a path that I can take with ease. I do not know how the cells would have been affected if instead of chemo they had been subjected to the attrition that can be caused by an estranged relationship. In any case, I would have had to overcome it alone.

Understanding the world of doctors

Doctors are often criticized for their inability to empathize with their patients, to listen to them, or to express themselves compassionately. We not only expect them to cure us, but to treat us with consideration and tact during the process. Almost without wishing to, we put them on a pedestal and we believe they have powers that they really don't have. Their word carries more weight than that of any one else's.

The fact that they coexist with illness and disease makes them neither omnipotent nor superior. They are humans like us, with their shortcomings and weaknesses.

A medical degree is one of the longest university degrees. In Spain, after six years of work, students are obliged to take en extremely tough exam, known as the MIR, in order to be able to specialize. They don't always pass, and if they do, their grade is often not high enough for them to specialize in their field of choice. So they end up specializing in something different from that which prompted them to study medicine in the first place. They go on to spend three years working as residents, or 'apprentices', in a hospital, but they often spend more hours at work than fully qualified physicians. They earn a salary, of course, but not enough to live on. And at the end of those three years, they may find themselves unemployed. When they finally obtain a position, which is not always where or what they want, they often have to move to another city. Reality does not always match up to what they imagined when they set out on their degree.

Their profession is characterized by a lack of time and resources to do their work as they would like and by the pressure they experience. They live under the constant threat of malpractice lawsuits a patient may present. To avoid this, doctors and oncologists collaborate in teams. They meet in committees to evaluate cases and share the decision-making. To safeguard their decisions and their involvement and to avoid lawsuits or defend themselves against them, they choose to follow a scheduled protocol. If they follow a protocol, their chances of being sued are much lower.

Protocols are standard procedures based on a number of variables. They are established after multiple studies on many patients. Each tumour, depending on the features described in Chapter 1 (size, location, progression, composition, hormonal sensitivity, etc.), that a doctor finds in a breast has its own scheduled treatment that has been tested in thousands of people and provided satisfactory results. The protocols are defined by the top hospitals in the field in question, the ones that are leading research and defining lines of action. In the case of breast cancer, the Hospital Vall d'Hebron, in Barcelona, is an international point of reference upheld by other institutions when applying treatments. Today, when we hear about personalized treatment of tumours, what it really means is that some highly specific protocols for action have been developed. Many different tumour classifications have been defined, each with a particular treatment, and, depending on the type of tumour, the relevant protocol is applied.

It is not a personalized treatment, as people are left out, excluded. The protocol takes precedence over the patient, whose sole power is to decide whether or not to take part in the established regimen by signing a consent. Any changes that the patient might want to propose will not be taken into account. Because what would happen if you opened that door?

Suppose a patient were to ask his doctor to ignore the protocol and change the treatment. And imagine the doctor agreed. If as a result the patient suffered after-effects, or died, and the family decided to sue, the doctor would not have a leg to stand on for not having followed the established protocol.

When the patient suffers these same after-effects but your doctor has followed the protocol to the letter, litigation is far less likely to succeed. But if he fails to follow protocols, not even a consent form rejecting the proposed treatment, signed by the patient, would protect the doctor in a court of law.

So, the doctor often has little leeway in the decision-making. If the protocol does not dictate the treatment, the rest of the medical team does. These professionals live in constant fear that the situation will turn against them. They cannot act as they would wish, because the consequences of possible errors could be very serious, and therefore they are forced to live with the frustration of not being able to do what they want.

Further to this, they may have a bad day; perhaps they have not overcome the death of a loved one which led them into the medical professional; or they have just had a problem with the previous patient, and this has affected them emotionally. We must remember that doctors see at least ten different people a day, so they cannot afford to get too close to their patients; and also what we consider to be serious to us is a daily occurrence to them; so downplaying treatment, creating distance, lacking empathy and evading the proposal of dialogue requested by the patient are easier to understand.

This is neither good nor bad. Doctors largely distance themselves due to their circumstances. They will be the first to defend the importance with which their training has taught them to deal with patient, to give the news, something that is no longer taught in Spanish universities. So given the circumstances, the doctors do as well as they can, resorting to a few short utterances, a tried and tested speech because that is what makes them feel secure. After several months of regular visits to the hospital for appointments or treatment, I can understand the burden of working every day in such a place. The sadness enveloping it can cast a shadow over anyone, and if you do not take care to detach yourself and turn a blind eye to the drama, you may find yourself drawn in too deeply.

We yearn for doctors to look us in the face, to know us, to know how to talk to us. We would like them to give over some of their time so they might see that we are different from the last patient who has just left their office, that we are more or less mature, more or less educated. I think it's a legitimate desire and a goal that we shouldn't give up, yet it is true that this is very complicated because everything – not just medicine – has become dehumanized. A lawyer you go to see about a problem will help you solve the case, but he will not cross the line between the professional and the personal relationship. It's easier, faster, and more convenient to keep the conversation at a level that requires the least involvement. It wards off fatigue, and a different attitude may even displease the customer, because that's not what he or she expects.

What sets apart the doctor-patient relationship from other established professional relationships is that the doctor is dealing with our health, a matter that is close to our hearts. Furthermore, it is an unequal relationship, because we only have one oncologist, one radiologist and so on, but they have many patients and therefore they cannot contribute the same dynamic to the relationship that the patient brings to them. They need to establish mechanisms to protect their intimacy against a person who bares his or hers, hence the barriers. Otherwise personal and emotional fatigue would wear them out.

You want to be a mother? Cryopreservation and other issues to consider

When a tumour appears at an age when one of your life projects is to raise a family, chemotherapy treatment presents an obstacle. Still, it's important to know there are options. A breast tumour does not close the door on fertility and motherhood.

As explained in Chapter 1, which describes tumour types and phases, a large number of tumours are hormone-dependent. This means that, to some extent, they 'feed' on female hormones and therefore, according to the traditional doctor's reasoning, it is best to halt female hormone production to avoid a relapse. Fortunately, this is no longer widely accepted in the scientific community. Today some allopathic physicians (those of the school of Western medicine) prefer not to cease the production of the hormone progesterone.

My tumour was extremely sensitive to hormones. How could it not be! If, as I believe, it was the result of a number of traumatic experiences over previous years, and characterized by hormonal insanity, the body necessarily reacts in some way.

During our interview with the doctor who gave me my diagnosis, I expressed my desire to have children. So I was referred to the gynecologic oncology department, which was launching a new technique called cryopreservation. Cryopreservation is designed to preserve ovarian tissue.

Before delving into a full-blown description of the procedure, I should clarify that, instead of undergoing surgery to remove ovarian tissue, it would be much simpler to remove eggs from the patient and freeze them prior to starting chemotherapy. I requested this procedure but was told there was no time (that urgency, once again) and,

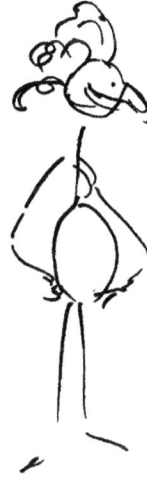

furthermore, they did not want to undergo hyperstimulation. Pilot studies conducted in 2009[8] suggest that it is possible to obtain viable oocytes in about ten or twelve days from the time you start treatment, without needing to wait for a new menstrual cycle. I don't know the impact that this stimulation might have on my body, but I find it hard to believe that ten days and a few hormones could cause a radical development of the tumour.

Returning to the subject of ovarian cryopreservation, the video found at the web address below describes the process:

http://myoncofertility.org/animations/ovarian_tissue_cryopreservation_basics

Laparoscopic surgery (a minimally invasive technique for accessing the desired organ through three or four small incisions) enables the surgeon to reach the ovaries. Once inside, the surgeon extracts some ovary tissue that is cut into thin sections called cortical strips that will be first analyzed to ensure they are healthy. If so, the strips are frozen for future use. Once the tumour has been treated (with chemo, radio, etc.) if the reproductive system has been affected and does not work properly, the frozen strips can be implanted into the patient's body so it can once again produce eggs.

My laparoscopy was painful. It's true that four small incisions are made, one of them at the navel, another at each ovary, and one more on the left side, below the ovary. But in my case, since they had already opened me up, the surgeon took advantage to remove a couple of fibroids (benign cysts on the uterine wall) and thus prevent potential problems in a future pregnancy. Perhaps this is why I felt so much pain during the postoperative period.

I went into the operating theatre on a Friday. I'd already had my first chemo session. The operation lasted about two hours. I was immediately awoken and put into a room with a female patient.

---

8. Source: "Ovarian stimulation to cryopreserve fertilized oocytes in cancer patients can be started in the luteal phase" von Wolff M, Thaler CJ, Frambach T, Zeeb C, Lawrenz B, Popovici RM, Strowitzki T. Fertility and Sterility 2009. www.fertstert.org/article/S0015-0282(08)03367-0/abstract

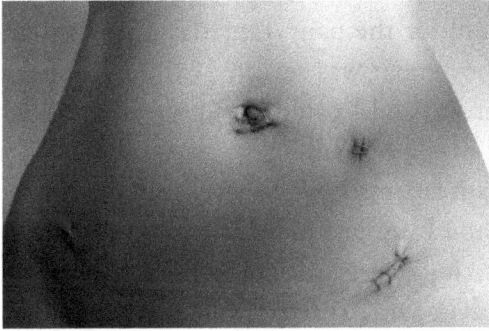

Laparoscopy

They ask you to get out of bed as soon as you can, the next day if possible, to get the bloodstream and kidneys working. My belly hurt when I got up! Then I had to take a shower. It was important to wash the surgical wounds. I did it myself (that's me). As I washed my hair, which I had had cut short, clumps began to fall out as a result of the chemotherapy. It was an unfortunate coincidence because I was not at my best physically or psychologically. I felt particularly embarrassed. I was sharing the room and shower, and I couldn't leave it in this state, with hair everywhere. So I bent down and pick it up with tissues. Writing about it now, I know it sounds ridiculous. I was in a hospital, in the oncology ward, surrounded by nurses and staff. My family was also there. I don't know how it could have occurred to me, in my condition, to bend over. I think between the anesthesia and the chemo I was a little 'stoned'. My mind wasn't functioning normally, and I was unable to reason properly. You become more sensitive and your emotions overwhelm you. At that point, the embarrassment I felt was much stronger than my common sense.

Moving around did not induce any complications; I was in agony, nothing more. But those moments are etched in my memory. My stay in the hospital was short. Two days later I was home. When you are discharged, you think you've made it through the most difficult time, and from there on your recovery will be quick and the pain will gradually subside. This didn't happen in my case. I was prescribed only paracetamol for the pain. One day I sneezed and felt a sharp twinge. Any movement was torture. I thought of the women who undergo a cesarean, and I couldn't fathom why nobody had warned me how bad it would be. But I understand that it's not the same for everyone. Perhaps laparoscopy really is a minimally invasive and painless technique and I was just unlucky for whatever reason, or was too optimistic, thinking that a little cut in the tummy would be nothing. Just in case, I advise you to prepare yourselves for a couple of difficult weeks. When you're young, people say you'll make a fast recovery and I believed it.

Once chemotherapy has been completed, no steps can be taken regarding pregnancy until a certain period of time has passed. This is to give the body time to eliminate any toxins that may have built up and to let it recover its normal functioning. After chemotherapy, there are several alternatives to become pregnant:

1. *Spontaneous Method*
   It's very important to wait at least one year from the last chemotherapy session before attempting pregnancy, even if your menstrual cycle has returned or you have not lost it. Your body is full of heavy metals that can cause fetal malformation.

2. *Ovarian hyperstimulation*
   Sometimes the ovaries work but they are weak. They are lazy and they need a nudge to wake them up. To this end, the patient needs daily injections of hormones in the tummy. For women with hormone-dependent breast cancer, specific treatments have been developed that are compatible with our clinical course. After hyperstimulation, a regular in vitro fertilization (IVF) process is initiated, whereby the eggs are removed, fertilized in the laboratory (normally using the partner's sperm) and one to three embryos are transferred back into

the patient's uterus, depending on how many have prospered and their quality.

3. Natural cycle IVF

This new but largely unknown technique has been successfully applied for many years in Japan, Switzerland and the United States. It relies on the single egg that our body produces in each cycle. After carrying out exhaustive hormonal monitoring, through a blood test, the patient is given a series of mild medications that induce egg maturity. The doctor has a four-hour window in which to puncture and remove the egg that is 'at its peak'. Afterwards, the IVF is performed. The great advantages of this method compared to ovarian hyperstimulation are that:

- It's a natural method that conforms to the natural evolution of our body's ovulation cycle. Ovarian hyperstimulation calls for the administration of high doses of artificial hormones that may have side effects.
- The puncture performed to remove the egg does not usually require anesthesia, and it is completed in a single puncture. Ovarian hyperstimulation seeks to collect as many eggs as possible, sometimes up to twenty, each one with its respective puncture. Hence the need for anesthesia.
- The monitoring of the process is simple, through blood tests.
- It's cheaper. The medications used cost a tenth of those for ovarian hyperstimulation.
- The implantation of a single egg avoids multiple pregnancies.
- As the procedure is non-invasive, you can try it over again.

Natural cycle IVF has proven effective in women for whom other options have failed. There is a specific technique of natural cycle IVF aimed at older women, or those with poor ovarian reserve, a common situation following chemotherapy.

4. *Egg donation*
Our body normally maintains the ability to gestate a fetus. If your hospital does not offer this option, there are ova banks and clinics specializing in this type of fertilization treatment.

5. *Reimplantation of ovarian tissue*
This is the latest option, the latest technology, the most laborious, the slowest and the least tested. But it has worked in several cases and over time the procedures will certainly improve and yield better results.

Normally you are recommended to try at least one of the first three options before resorting to the reimplantation of ovarian tissue, because it is still in the experimental phase and has a low success rate. If you do choose reimplantation, you'll find it a fascinating process. Before I was explained how it worked, I assumed the reimplantation would be performed in the same place from where the samples were extracted at the time, from the ovary. I was wrong. There are several methods by which the implant can be performed. But the one I was told about at the time, and that really caught my attention, involves implanting the tissue in the forearm! Yes, that's right. They make some small cuts and transplant it. Then it's a question of waiting to see if the grafted tissue 'attaches' and the technique works or not. It can be likened to planting a cutting. The tissue needs nourishment so it creates capillaries by which to receive this nourishment. Sometimes it does not have enough strength to revive and mature the eggs it contains. And sometimes it does. So your eggs are removed and thus begins the fertilization process that today is so common.

Nevertheless, although various options to facilitate pregnancy after chemotherapy are being investigated and tested, their approach will not always get the approval of oncologists. Normally, the protocol for a hormone-dependent tumour requires the patient to take tamoxifen for five years. This tablet is taken once daily and is incompatible with pregnancy. We will examine this subject in more depth in the next chapter.

In my case, I do not know if it is because I'd had a failed pregnancy when they discovered the tumour, because I was trying to get pregnant again, because I like to question everything, or because I cannot accept impositions that are beyond common sense, the fact is I take a rather critical stance with respect to hormonal suppression.

I had the good fortune to have a chat with an expert physician in this field who inspires total confidence in me. After listening to my story she encouraged me to get pregnant as soon as possible because, according to her, pregnancy itself inhibits the development of new tumours. She represents a current school of thought and a work style that does not fit the usual protocols in Spain, but it works (and very well) in other countries.

I began chemotherapy in October and had my last period in November. I finished chemo the following April. I was thirty-seven years old. I thought my period would come again right away, but it didn't. It took almost a year! At first I didn't understand why a friend of mine – quite a bit older than I and who hadn't wanted children – had regained her period after a couple of months, and why for me it was taking so long. Six months after the chemo I went to see the gynecologic oncologist who had performed the laparoscopy. When he saw my analyses he said, with that tact so typical of some professionals, "You're menopausal …" It was like a slap in the face, so inconsiderate. Luckily by then I knew this type of doctor and was prepared for any bad news. I replied that my menstrual cycle could still return, that my body could still awaken, that it was readjusting. He replied, his voice incredulous, that anything can happen in medicine, but thought it unlikely.

Curiously, I had gone to this appointment alone. And I was struck by my own reaction and detachment at his comment. I honestly did not believe what he said. It seemed to me that with this reply he merely sought to protect himself, to be on the safe side. But I didn't throw in the towel, or let it get to me. I left there thinking "He'll see that my body reacts".

And indeed, it did! It didn't take much longer. My period came two months later. When I returned to see the gynecologist who had declared me 'menopausal', he was no longer there, he had retired. The doctor who greeted me clearly formed part of a new generation and a new way of doing things. She was lovely and encouraged me to get pregnant in a few months.

One last thing, before starting

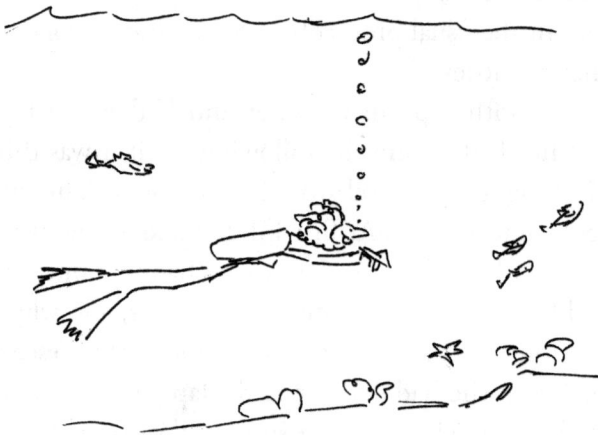

Once we saw that there was a possibility (the slimmest of slim chances) that the analysis of my lump would test positive, we went on holiday. We had ten days from the time we delivered the biopsy to the hospital to the day of the results. So after handing in the little treasure we went straight to a travel agency. It was early August. The whole process had begun in July, when I visited my family doctor to show her my little lump, and from there to the gynecologist, thereafter to the radiologist, and lastly having the ultrasound and biopsy. So we let some time transpire without making any concrete plans for the August holidays. After the battery of tests, we decided to get away towards the end of the month, do some scuba diving and relax in sun loungers. We were naïve! We thought that all this would end after the results, but it was only just beginning.

The doctor who did the biopsy took advantage of a moment when I went to the bathroom to make it clear to Joss that the sooner we left for vacation the better. Upon our return, we would get the results.

Further testing was carried out to identify the type and size of the tumour. Once we learned the final diagnosis, I was referred to an oncologist. During this time we were still able to make several weekend getaways to hike in the mountains. I sensed what lay in store, so over that month I began to take better care of myself. I exercised more, ate healthier food, tried to build up my strength and did more research. It was around this time I met Master Jin and that I visited the homeopath from whose office I fled aghast. I bought some books, and I promised myself that cancer, as everyone called it, would not be part of our daily dinner table conversation. Everything comes to an end, and we would surmount the stages of treatment little by little, step by step, I thought. But we would not allow the tumour to become the sole topic of conversation. Life goes on, and many things continue to happen around you. As you withdraw somewhat from the world, your friends and your family are doing things, and feeling things, living fascinating experiences to which you can connect, and also experience through them.

My negotiations with the oncologist began from day one. When I went to find out the type of chemotherapy I would have, he wanted to set a starting date for the first cycle (as they call each session), but Joss and I didn't agree. We said we weren't ready yet, we needed a week (I don't recall if Joss had to travel, or simply if we had a few things pending that we wanted to resolve). This was, and remains, the tone of my relationship with the oncologist. He proposes and together we discuss and reach a consensus. He is an approachable man who doesn't change his position easily (sometimes the negotiations are arduous, and I don't always have my way). He really gives the best of himself.

Chapter Four

CONVENTIONAL TREATMENTS

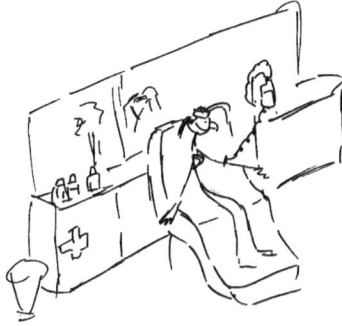

As we have seen, there are many different types of tumours, some bigger, some smaller, some more sensitive to hormones, some less so. Before proposing and beginning a treatment, the doctors carefully study all these parameters to find the most effective way to attack the cancer cells. That said, there is something we all undergo, and that's surgery. Some women have radiotherapy, chemotherapy, hormone therapy. And certainly there are more types of treatments. I will speak only of those I know, and in general terms. My tumour was one of the most common types (which develop in 80% of women), so at least we will cover a wide range of women with tumours.

Which is the first treatment?

Depending on the urgency and the types of tumour, the doctor will choose surgery or chemotherapy as the first step. Radiotherapy is always left for later, to finish cleaning any microscopic tumour cell debris that might have remained.

Things to consider

If the tumour is small or has already spread to the lymph nodes, the doctors often choose to operate first. Usually they attempt to conserve the breast, a procedure known as breast-conserving surgery or lumpectomy. Depending on the severity and extent of the tumour, a mastectomy may be performed in which the entire breast is removed.

In addition to removing the tumour, during surgery the surgeons remove the sentinel lymph node under the arm that is on the same side where the tumour is located, and analyze it then and there in the operating theatre. If the node is clean, they don't touch anything else. The surgeons close the incisions and give you a few weeks to recover before continuing. If the node is affected, they remove the entire cluster of axillary lymph nodes to ensure that no cancer cells remain in the body.

If the tumour is large (more than 5 cm in diameter), the doctors may opt for chemotherapy first, in order to shrink it and thus avoid having to remove the whole breast.

My case fell within the second group: large and not very aggressive. Moreover, the lymph nodes were not affected.

It is important, or at least it was until recently, to point out how decisive the order of the treatments can be. Here's what I mean: I had two scans and two biopsies, and even a nodal ultrasound, before any decision was made on how to approach my treatment. The doctors needed to collect more data because my diagnosis was unclear. On the one hand, it seemed that the tumour was quite large but, on the other, the lymph nodes did not appear to be affected, and these two things proved to be contradictory within the protocol classifications of cancer medicine (see Chapter 1, 'Tumour types and phases'). I was convinced that the lymph nodes were not affected. Master Jin, an expert practitioner of TCM, also ensured me this was the case. So I had no objection when I was proposed to undergo chemotherapy before surgery, to see if it would shrink the tumour, and this way conserve the breast.

What I was not told then is that while the sentinel lymph node is a reliable test before chemotherapy, it is not considered as such afterwards. Doctors say that treatment can affect the drainage channels and therefore, although the sentinel lymph node may come out clean, it is still possible that the disease may have spread to other nodes. So if I had been operated before the chemotherapy, the surgeons would not have removed the cluster of lymph nodes, only the sentinel. With surgery as a second step, the sentinel lymph node biopsy is no longer reliable; consequently my lymph nodes were removed. The chapter on lymphedema examines the importance of the lymph nodes and the lymphatic system, and the risks associated with lymph node removal. But it is important to understand from the outset the importance of the order of decisions. A minor initial intervention (which they neither offered nor discussed with me) to remove and analyze the sentinel lymph node prior to beginning the process would have yielded reliable information that probably would have avoided such aggressive surgery and consequent after-effects.

What happened in my case? At the end of chemotherapy I went to see my doctor – the same who once gave me the diagnosis and then prescribed the chemo first and operation after – to discuss the surgery, and I was stunned to hear her say matter-of-factly that my lymph nodes would have to be removed.

I was not given a choice. I had just completed my eighth cycle of chemo. It had not been four weeks since the last cycle. I was still psychologically optimistic, but powerless to argue as I would have if the discussion took place today.

That day, the conversation did not actually start on that note, it was even worse: Joss and I had been waiting some while. We had come to learn the results after chemotherapy. We knew they were very good, that the tumour had shrunk from 5.5 cm to less than 1 cm. So we had managed to save the breast. Furthermore, the lymph node ultrasound had confirmed that they were fine. So we were ready for the next step, knowing that the worst was behind us.

The doctor came into the office, and almost without looking us in the eye, said: "We'll have to remove the breast because there are some small spots that could be malignant nodules, and, just in case, it'd be better to remove it."

After much give and take attempts to speak the same language as the doctor, Joss – who was the most lucid of the three – suggested an exploratory surgery, after which a sample could be analyzed and – in case anything remained – a second operation could be performed. But not remove the entire breast all at once with "just in case" as a justification. What I found and still find astonishing is that the doctor agreed. My conclusion was that if the patient is strong, logical, and has the capacity to fight for her breast, she will save it; but if not, if you are weak, without sound arguments, they will remove it.

What kind of criterion is that?

Having saved my breast, after half an hour of discussion, we turned to the matter of the lymph nodes. The doctor said without flinching that they would have to be removed, *just in case* (again). I offered to sign a paper exempting her from any liability in the event that the tumour should reappear, or should lymph nodes become affected. And I expressed openly, and repeatedly, that I did not want them removed. She replied it was either that or nothing. And pretty much dismissed us.

Before the operation, we made another appointment with the same doctor, for we could not believe there was nothing else that could be done, that we did not have the right, as the directly affected people, to decide what we wanted.

What right does a doctor have to decide what is better or worse for me, and who imposes an ultimatum, rather than look at me in the face and give me alternatives? From where does he or she acquire this omnipotence that I have not afforded her? Did the doctor decide out of fear of a subsequent lawsuit? I was willing to sign an exemption of liability, whatever was necessary, and even so, it could not be. She didn't come to the appointment we had asked for prior to the surgery. She avoided all personal responsibility and sent someone from her staff instead.

Of everything I've been through over the last two years, of all the people I have met, all the conversations I have taken part in and decisions I've been making, of all these experiences, this is my most bitter memory. I have had a hard time overcoming the resentment and anger towards this person who is not even aware of what her actions have meant to me, simply for not taking the time to listen. To her mind, what's done has been done well because she has saved lives no matter if it has been done insensitively.

My rage at this decision was exacerbated when two things happened: the first, and which I recount in the chapter on after-effects, is that I developed lymphedema in my arm. Surely this would not have happened but for the removal of the lymph nodes. The second is that several months after the operation I read a medical paper in which my own doctor explained how, in cases like mine, the protocol has since been modified due to the findings of a study conducted by her team, from which they were able to deduce that sentinel lymph node biopsy continued to be reliable after chemotherapy. Incidentally, these studies had already been conducted in other hospitals, where the protocol I have just described has been implemented for years.

In defence of our rights

We may think we are entitled to have an opinion and to have the right to be treated with respect. While we don't hold a degree in Medicine, we are people who are capable of making our own decisions. My doctors chose to ignore me to avoid risks, without looking at me, without taking me into account. And it would have been much more satisfying for everyone to have listened to me, for if I'm wrong about what concerns me – and I consider myself qualified and informed enough to decide – no one should question or change my decisions.

Some of you will surely be wondering if I ended up signing the authorization that would allow them to operate on me. Of course I did! But under what conditions? After eight cycles of chemotherapy, an hour of conversation with the doctors, and the clear message that this is how things work in this hospital, take it or leave it. In all honesty, I'm not saying I signed under duress, but I let the reader draw their own conclusions. Perhaps there was the option to change hospitals, to find another doctor. But when one can barely climb ten steps in a row because of exhaustion, to undertake such a search is a difficult and complicated task.

Aware of the difficulties in the doctor-patient relationship, and of the existing social debate around this, some years back politicians began work on drawing up the current legislation regarding the rights of patients. There are regional, national and international laws and decrees. Moreover, the joint efforts of groups and associations have also made headway along the same lines. One major contribution to this end was made in 2003, when patient associations met in Barcelona to discuss the vision and experience of patients in six areas of interest:

- Information needs of patients.
- Patient involvement in clinical decision-making.
- Communication and doctor-patient relationship and communication.
- Patient accessibility to health care.
- Patient involvement in health policy.
- Patients' rights.

The conclusions reached at this meeting can be found on the Internet (see bibliography). In addition, the associations drafted a 'Decalogue of patients' (see Annex 1), which brings the social debate into focus and reflects a growing concern to involve patients in decision-making and respect their judgement. This annex also includes the WMA (World Medical Association) Declaration of Lisbon on the Rights of the Patient, adopted in October 1981 and finally revised in October 2005.

In 2006, P. Simon,[9] Professor at the Andalusian School of Public Health published an article in Spanish entitled 'Ten myths about informed consent.' In these ten pages, Simon provides a thorough analysis of the current situation of patients. He takes into account the law and draws some accurate conclusions that give some food for thought.

❖ Clinicians alone can no longer know what consists of 'doing good' for the patient. The patient's opinion is essential, without it there are no correct clinical actions.

❖ Today, the good surgeon – by way of an example – is not just a professional who operates well; he or she also provides patients with quality information, involves them in decision-making and obtains valid consent.

❖ Patients will need fewer clinicians to obtain scientific information because the Internet is already providing this [...]. Thus, the key role of the health professional of the future will not be to seek scientific information, but to provide advice and assistance in the process of clinical decision-making.

While it's true that more and more voices are being raised on this issue and seeking the best way to implement the legislation, through workshops and specific training aimed at healthcare professionals, in

9. SIMON, P. (2006), "Diez mitos en torno al consentimiento informado" ["Ten myths about informed consent"], *Anales* journal, vol. 29, Suppl. 3. "La relación clínica en el siglo XXI". Pp 29-40. Anales del Sistema Sanitario de Navarra. Published by the Department of Health of the Autonomous Government of Navarre.

practice it's clear that much remains to be done. Consequently, the health service, the patient and even the doctor (the party most satisfied with the results of their work) would benefit from its implementation, which is still far from standard procedure.

Chemotherapy

Chemotherapy consists of the administration, usually intravenously, of a set of drugs. Full treatment consists of several sessions, each called a 'cycle'. In the case of a breast tumour, cycles are administered every three weeks. Chemotherapy drugs are characterized by their extreme aggression. They are complex of chemicals agents designed to attack and kill tumour cells. The direct consequence of the application of chemotherapy and the reason the treatment has such a bad reputation is because it generates significant side effects that greatly reduce the patient's quality of life for the duration of the process, and in many cases, once it has been completed.

In truth, chemotherapy is a 'fix' that leaves you half-drugged and your body in rather bad shape. Small wonder its bad reputation. But I don't wish to enter into the debate about this type of treatment. As we have seen, sometimes how and why you do something is more important. There are detractors of chemotherapy who speak of it as if it were a poison; indeed, it really does attack the entire body, and it is hard to believe that something that causes so many harmful effects can be good. Obviously, chemotherapy also has its advocates; those who are not happy with the side effects but believe that it is the best available treatment to date to destroy tumours and cancer cells.

Many people contend that chemotherapy was invented by the big pharmaceutical companies to make money. The products used are very expensive, and the pharmaceutical industry has become a very powerful force in the world. It has pressure groups (lobbies) in different national and international organizations that try to influence decision-making and the drafting of laws to suit their interests. The example of the malaria or caries vaccines are well known, which after their discovery are not being sold because their use would result in huge financial losses that these companies currently earn through the sales of their healing remedies. This is a subject of current debate. It's worth mentioning, although we will not examine it in depth in this book.

* * *

I considered bypassing chemotherapy and seeking an alternative way to deal with the tumour. In the end I chose to have it, in addition to other solutions that I will discuss later. What is clear is that after everything I've done, if any cells still floundered, with the onslaughts they received on all fronts, they must have got to a better place.

For my part, I feel at ease. I am certain that I have done, and continue to do, everything in my power to change the patterns that caused the tumour in the first place. I have done everything in which I believe. If you search the Internet, you will always find statistics to justify everything, which can only instil more and more fear. One day, while casually browsing some blogs, I came upon a study claiming that women who drank alcohol moderately were more likely to relapse.

Well, how do you feel after reading that? Do you stop having a glass of wine with your dinner if that's what you like? Don't the experts say that a glass of good quality red wine is highly beneficial for many things? If you stop drinking, stop eating, stop breathing the pollution in cities, stop experiencing strong emotions that can cause stress, become pregnant early, or not, better late (depending on the study), stop using salt, living a hectic life and so on. If we leave all that out by necessity, maybe we would forget to live.

I have been adapting my daily life to a new situation from everything I've learned, and it's true I don't eat meat, I consume less salt and no refined flour and try to eat organic products. But I still do and will continue to have a glass of wine when I want, and I keep thinking about getting pregnant at some point. Because that's what my inner voice tells me, what I believe, and what I'm committed to.

Things to consider

Should I have a portacath placed?

The portacath is a catheter, a tube that is inserted under the skin and allows direct access to one of the large central veins of our body to administer medication.

Chemotherapy is so aggressive that it affects some of the large veins. They are exposed directly to the agents, which eventually cause them to lose flexibility, become fragile and deteriorate in general, especially if the port is in the arm, as its veins are relatively thin compared to central veins. Moreover, this being far from the heart, the medication does not reach the rest of the body directly, but must first go up the arm and into the heart to be distributed through the body. To mitigate these effects and prevent wear on the blood vessels, it is possible to implant a portacath.

This device is a catheter the size of a large round button. It is inserted in the operating theatre, under local anesthesia, and is located

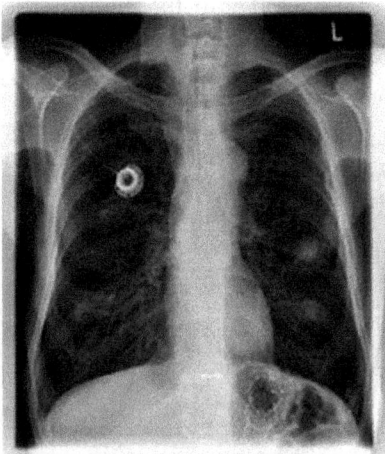

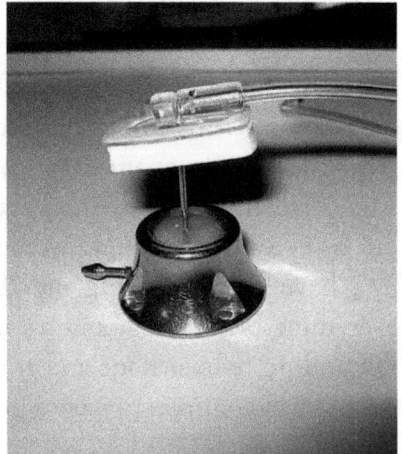

under the skin, more or less at the neckline, on the side opposite from the tumour (to not interfere with surgery). A subcutaneous tube also runs from this 'button' up to the neck until it disappears into one of our large veins. Treatment is administered by pricking the centre of the 'button', which can be felt with the fingers.

This is one of the first decisions to make before starting chemotherapy, or sometimes after the first session: whether you want to have a catheter placed or if you prefer to have the chemo administered in the arm, as it is usually done in the hospital with saline and medicines through a tube.

My first big fight took place in the operating theatre when I was to have the portacath inserted. I got very worked up in an attempt to defend my cleavage. I didn't want to have a visible scare there. In all my thirty-five years I had never entered an operating theatre, and within months, I had already amassed five scars and there were still three more to come. Between us women, I still have trouble accepting the scar left by the portacath whenever I see it, but over time its outline has faded.

Beyond that, the process seemed simple. You are given an appointment and, in an outpatient procedure, you lie on a trolley and are wheeled into the operating room. After a couple of hours you're back home with your portacath installed.

The first time I was scheduled, I had just received my first cycle of chemo the day before. You are asked not to eat for six hours prior to the procedure, so there I was, on 28 September 2009, with all my best intentions, my aching body and my nausea.

You are explained the surgical procedure and the type of anesthesia you will be given as you are being prepared. Then they put a sedative under your tongue to keep you calm and tell you about some activities that are incompatible with the catheter. This is when the alarm bells sounded. I was wearing the cap, clad in the robe, lying on the trolley with paper booties on, the sedative in my mouth, when I was told I would not be able to practise scuba diving. Red alert! We had not been warned about this! And you're supposed to keep the portacath in place for five years (according to protocol, once again, since you don't get the official all-clear until five years after the tumour was first diagnosed). The fact is that both the nurse and the doctor were superb, for Joss and I refused to have a device installed that would prevent me from diving for five years. If they tell you to live a normal life, and my normal life involves going on a diving holiday somewhere at least once a year, this was hard to accept.

So, we decided to discuss the dates with the oncologist. If he agreed to remove the portacath after the chemo, I would return and have the catheter placed.

I dressed and we went home, high on the sedative and in shock from the information. The other activity incompatible with the port-acath is hunting, which I couldn't care less about because I don't go in for that sport.

My understanding is that this was the first time someone had left the operating theatre for personal reasons rather than clinical incom-patibilities.

The second attempt took place on Monday October 19th. On the morning of that day I had been to see my oncologist for the first check-up and to set the day for my second chemo cycle, theoretically for the next day. It would have been three weeks since the first cycle. But during this interval I had had the laparoscopy to remove ovarian tissue, so my defences were rather low and the treatment was post-poned for another week.

Once again, on an empty stomach, I relaxed as much as I could on the trolley. I could barely move because of the pain from the laparos-copy. It took a supreme effort to lie down and get up. But there we were: Joss stayed with me while I donned the cap, the paper booties, the robe and the blanket. And we waited... And waited... And wait-ed... The surgeon arrived, five hours later, to apologize because he'd had to deal with an emergency case with complications and had sev-eral other patients waiting. So for the second time we returned home without the portacath, but with a date set for the next attempt.

At the third attempt (the Wednesday of that same week), I had the portacath installed.

You're awake in the operating theatre. You see nothing, because your face is covered with a sheet. The only part of your body that is exposed is the area of the incision. And I did nothing but plead with the surgeons to make the cut lower down, so it would not be noticeable, I wanted to keep my cleavage unblemished. I imagine it was thanks to my insistence because the surgeon went to great pains, and to close the wound he used the same technique as the one used in cosmetic surgery.

You can probably all imagine a freshly stitched wound, where the stitches or staples go from one side to the other. After a few days, they are removed and the healing continues. The technique to which I refer, and which is also used in cosmetic surgery, differs slightly. Stiches are also used, but they are internal; that is, they are placed under the skin at a deeper level. Afterwards the wound is closed with so-called 'butterfly stitches' or 'Steri-Strips', which are actually very thin strips of adhesive bandage that are applied down the length of the wound (often also across the wound to pull either side of it together). After a few days, which may vary depending on what the doctor suggests, you can remove these strips yourself at home, with soap and water. The wound is now closed, and the only evidence is a thin line in the skin, without those pesky marks left by standard stitches, and without the overextension caused by badly connected layers of tissue.

My portacath protruded substantially. Especially as the months passed, as I was becoming all skin and bones. It was especially bothersome when I drove because it came into contact with the seatbelt, and when I was wearing a shoulder bag. Its presence was constant.

As soon as I finished the chemotherapy (I was still undergoing radiotherapy sessions), I asked for it to be removed. The nurses were surprised to learn that I had not had it in for even a year, until I made a comment and one nurse exclaimed, "Ah, you're the diver!" Clearly my case had been widely discussed. And exactly as we had agreed together with the doctors, I had the portacath removed without any problem. Yet again I had to go in several times because I wanted the same surgeon to do it, the one who used the 'invisible' sutures. He made a clean incision, and in a jiffy the 'thingy' was out. That was in July 2010. That summer I was able to dive.

Before your hair starts to fall out

Coping with and starting the whole process that revolves around the issue of hair loss was, for me, the hardest.

And I suppose most women who have had this experience will agree. The fact is that you look for a solution before the problem arises, before you see your hair fall out, and, of course, it takes a bit of getting used to the idea. I believe that's the first time one becomes aware of the process that awaits you. Deep down you entertain the hope that, like other more or less random side effects, it won't happen to you. But I don't think anyone can avoid it.

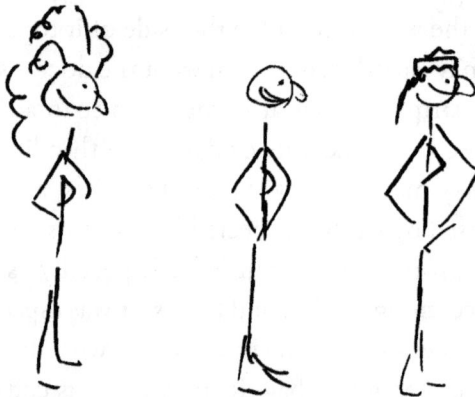

There are many specialized centres that offer a range of solutions. None of them convinced me because I didn't feel like I identified with them. Just as on my wedding day I didn't see myself wearing one of those cancan dresses, this time I couldn't see myself in a wig. Nor did I see myself wearing only a scarf. You expose yourself to many questions, you stand out in a crowd, and I was not prepared for that. I wanted to avoid being noticed at all costs, but I could not see how.

So I turned to a good friend who is a designer and stylist and she immediately came up with a solution. She understood me perfectly (she also helped me with my wedding style; she knows my tastes almost better than I do so she knew exactly what to suggest). She got in touch with a hairdresser friend who, like her, works in the media, and together they set to work.

We started by going to some wig shops. The first thing is to do is to rule out options. In order to make sure I didn't want a wig, we tried on a few to see how they looked on me, and if I felt comfortable. And I felt terrible! Some of my friends who have gone through the same experience have worn wigs, and the truth is they looked much better on them. A wig was definitely not for me.

These friends who helped me so much are stylists and work with wigs on a daily basis, creating characters, and they know how uncomfortable they can be. They itch, they make you feel hot, they easily come out of place, and they have to be handled with great care. And some people like doing this: combing the hair at night, taking it to be cleaned and so forth. But I don't even use a hairdryer in my daily life, and I am really lazy about having a haircut.

What did we do then? A genuine work of art.

First we bought some Buffs, also called a neck gaiter, a kind of headwear mainly used for alpine sports, to protect the neck or head. It is a seamless tube made of a high quality lightweight microfiber fabric, which is breathable and easy to wash. It can be worn in many ways, and in fact the Buff company has produced a booklet with instructions on how to wear Buffs, specifically for cancer patients (see Annex 4). As your hair falls out your head loses volume, and if you use only a Buff or scarf to cover baldness, your head will look disproportionately small. Hence the Buff company's proposal, get two: one for volume, and the second as a hat to wear on your head.

We did something different. We took a black Buff and folded it to make a cap. This would cover my scalp and provide a base upon which to add hair. My hairdresser friend bought some natural hair extensions in my colour and treated them. She dyed them a little to create some highlights, and sewed them around the cap. Then I tried it on and she trimmed the hair to make it resemble my own, always dishevelled and falling around my face. She left a space for my ears, and made a sideswept fringe. The hair she bought and styled looked very similar to mine, which is fine and wavy.

This was the first part of the process. With the base now complete, we played around with some accessories: hats, scarves, Buffs or neckerchiefs that I would wear on top of the 'cap'. I used different combinations; particularly other Buffs that I wore as scarfs. I had them in different colours; they were easy to wear, protected your head, and kept you warm without feeling confined or tight-fitting. In addition, they washed very easily. Even the hair extensions could be washed and combed easily.

I was lucky. That winter all kinds of caps, hats and berets were in vogue, and they lent themselves to many possibilities of styles. It was even fun. My designer friend and I got lost in stores trying on everything. And the hair extension passed an endless 'battery of tests'. Even the nurses thought it was my own and that I was wearing the cap or the Buff because it was fashionable. I looked at myself in the mirror and I looked great. One day, I amused myself on the underground counting the number of people who wore accessories on their head, and out of some twenty people I counted seven, myself included. It

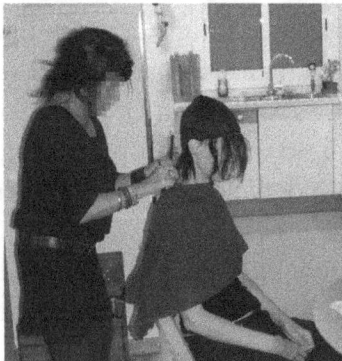

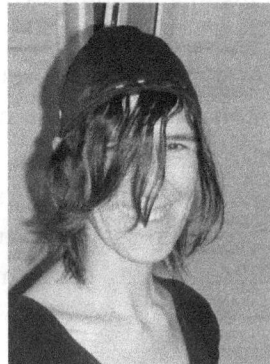

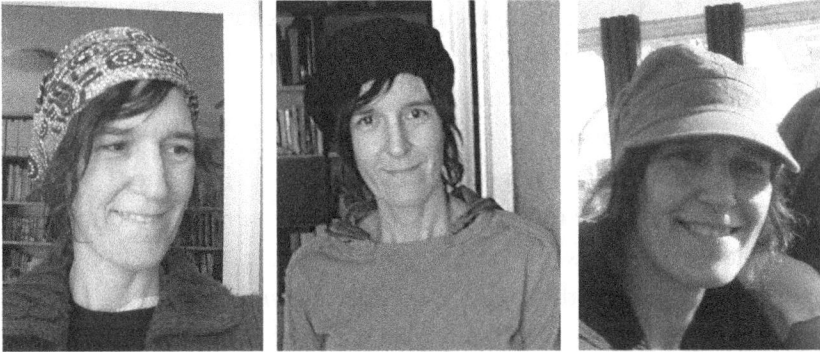

was hard to imagine the real reason why I was wearing mine, and this knowledge gave me peace of mind.

What's more, I could ride a motor scooter and wear the helmet without fear of being seen bald in the middle of the street! If I was wearing a beret, I would remove it, and I was visible for a couple seconds wearing the black cap, before I donned my helmet. No one noticed I was wearing something unusual on my head, because of the black cap. If I was wearing Buffs or a neckerchief, I put the motorbike helmet on directly over it. To take it off all I had to do was take care not to move the structure. I never found myself exposing my baldness to people, nor did I go through awkward situations that I know can make one feel vulnerable and helpless. So obviously I recommend my option, that's why I'm sharing it with you. Still, it's true that, like everything else, the important thing is to find the alternative that is best for each one of us.

I realize that not everyone knows someone who knows about hair extensions and wigs, or sometimes we don't feel like asking for help. If you fancy trying the option I have described, there is the alternative of buying ready-made fringes or half-wigs in specialized shops. They can be combined in the same manner as I did with my hair extensions, and are not as hot as a full wig.

If you choose to wear only scarves of the type that are sold in places specialized in solutions for cancer patients (how little I like these terms!) they will show you how to wear them. As I explained about the Buff, it's important to lend volume to the head. Sometimes we forget that the hair somehow enlarges the perception of the head. If we don't have hair and we cover our head it seems very small. So there are ways to wear neckerchiefs, scarves or Buffs to make the size of your head look more normal.

Lastly, the wig is another option. And there are thousands to choose from! They are made of natural hair, artificial hair, made to measure or by catalogue. Prices can vary, depending on the quality. After trying on a few to see how they felt, I was fully convinced they are not my thing. For this reason, I will only give it a brief mention. If you really want to try some you can get information at the abovementioned centres, or directly on the Internet.

The wig will never perfectly mirror your hair or your regular haircut, not even a custom-made wig of natural hair, although it may look more authentic than the artificial type. Before choosing a natural hair wig, I suggest you look at some ready-made ones. Given the cost of a natural wig it's important, and worthwhile to explore other alternatives.

Moreover, wigs often end up in the drawer. Some people cannot bear the texture of the fabric on their scalp. And it would be a shame to waste so much effort on something that finally doesn't fulfil your expectations.

Some women have taken this opportunity to completely change their image. And they put on a huge mane of blond hair, curly hair, dark hair... a look diametrically opposed to what they normally have. It's a good idea if you like to experiment.

Eyebrows and the rest of the face

Naturally, we don't only lose the hair on our head. Our eyebrows and the hair on the rest of our body hair slowly fall out. Some people conserve the hair in their armpits, sometimes not even that.

It's interesting to see how, after going bald, our eyebrows and eyelashes resist against all odds. There are cases of women whose facial hair didn't start to fall out until after completing chemotherapy. What is certain is that, like the hair on your head, your body hair will also fall out. This happens over time. Our eyebrows and eyelashes gradually thin out, so it's a good idea to prepare for this and have the necessary resources at hand, since losing this hair can be especially traumatic for some people because they lose their facial expression. We immediately perceive it, but it's one of those things that with a few tricks and some makeup can be hidden well. A good idea is to take a photo of yourself before your eyebrows begin to disappear, to have a reference on which to rely when they're gone.

The *micropigmentation* technique used to make tattoos may also be used to draw the shape of our eyebrows permanently. Many centres specializing in solutions for cancer patients often have access to this technique, as well as beauty centres that offer 'permanent makeup'. Regardless of the outcome, which will depend largely on the professional expertise, it's important to note that this technique consists of making tiny pinpricks on the skin to insert ink into the dermis. We know that chemotherapy lowers our defences and makes us more vulnerable to all manner of infections. So micropigmentation should be carried out before starting the chemo.

Another simpler and less expensive option is to put on makeup every day. One technique, which worked well for me, consists of first using a sharp brown pencil to draw the hairs, and then applying brown shadow as filler on the hairs drawn. This option allows you to replicate the shape and swirls of the brow, and the result looks quite natural. After a week you get used to it and can do it almost without thinking. There are also false eyebrows and templates that can be purchased in pharmacies or specialized beauty centres.

As the eyelashes also fall out, it never hurts to outline the eyes, at least the upper eyelid. In terms of colours, everyone has different tastes. But it can be interesting to go for a tone that softens the expression, such as browns, greys, blues and so forth.

The rest of the face would appreciate some extra moisturizing. Ideally, use natural products. Laboratory creams often contain parabens, which are synthetic chemicals derived from petroleum.[10] You can use natural oils, and even make a homemade unguent by mixing wheat germ oil with olive oil and macadamia nut oil in equal parts. To facilitate absorption and prevent excess oil, use rose water as a facial toner.

It's also advisable to protect your skin with a high factor sun cream. Chemotherapy causes photosensitivity, making our skin more prone to burning or to the appearance of blemishes. Lastly, a small amount of blusher and moisturizing lipstick will give us that shimmer that the skin loses.

Dentist appointment

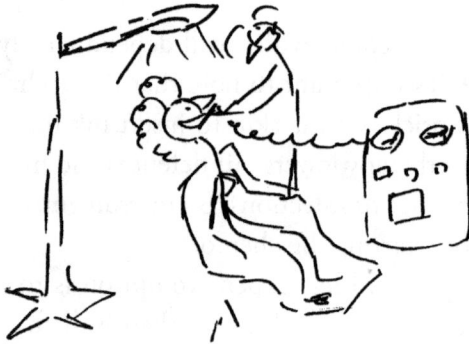

While you are undergoing chemotherapy it's best to avoid any other treatment that may favour the proliferation of infections. This includes dental cleaning, extractions and fillings. So it's best to check before starting the chemotherapy that your mouth is healthy and that you won't need treatment for a time. In addition, the gums and tooth

---

10. The discovery of parabens in a number of breast tumour samples has given rise to speculation that these molecules may travel from the armpit, where they are applied in deodorants, to the milk duct, thus contributing to the development of a tumour. Although I don't wish to engage in polemics, TCM frowns upon skin care products that cannot be ingested, since the skin also absorbs these products.

enamel may be affected by the chemo. Have a check-up beforehand to be able to later assess the impact of treatment.

Chemotherapy and its side effects

The first time I found myself in the queue to get into the day hospital I was overwrought, wondering what the coming year would bring, how my body would react, how I would feel. I felt a certain curiosity about a world to which I had always been oblivious. I had never been sick. My only stay in the hospital had been a year earlier, after having a miscarriage, due to an infection. The truth is, having this type of treatment and what would come afterwards is not something you include in your life map.

That doesn't stop it from being an incredible situation, a kind of adrenaline rush, thinking that henceforth, and until further notice, everything that will happen to you will be new, something never experienced. It reminds me of the feeling you get when you move to another city, country or start a new job, and you're wondering how the first day of your new life will be there, if you'll adapt, if the people will be nice, if you will like it. Well that's how I felt. I would rather have not had to go through it, of course, preferring they had never found the growth. But, once placed in that situation, I would experience it in the best way possible.

I entered a sunny and spacious room with friendly people and comfortable sofas. I could tell the nurses knew what they were doing, which gave me a sense of security. Apart from one patient taking delight in recounting her woes and tragedies for all to hear, the atmosphere was relaxed. You were welcomed to a place where you would be accompanied along the way, helped and made to feel as comfortable as possible. What wonderful people!

I sat on a sofa and listened to the explanation of the procedure. I hadn't even had the portacath placed yet, so the nurse connected me to a tube and began to deliver various liquids.

Breast chemotherapy typically combines two types of drugs. The standard procedure is to deliver six or eight cycles of chemotherapy, three and three, or four and four of each type of substance, consecutively. The first substance is easily recognizable by its red colour. It is commonly referred to as 'the red one'. It's a combination of doxorubicin (which gives it that colour) and cyclophosphamide. These drugs act on the tumour cells. When used as neoadjuvant or induction therapy, which is the kind applied before chemotherapy or radiotherapy, its objective is to halt the growth of the tumour and shrink it. When used as adjuvant therapy, i.e. after surgery, its purpose is to attack any remaining tumour cells in order to prevent the reproduction or spread of the tumour.

Each cycle of chemotherapy as such, meaning the time one spends in the hospital connected to a drip that is delivering the treatment, lasts about an hour and a half. You begin to feel the effect within ten minutes of starting. One good piece of advice I got from the nurses when I went to the hospital for my first treatment was to ignore what people tell you, because you won't necessarily experience the side effects that others do. Looking back I see they were absolutely right. The more you read and the more you hear makes you more aware of what you are supposed to experience, so I suggest you even skip this chapter on side effects and return to it only if necessary.

Straight away, from the moment you are connected to the drip, you start to feel groggy. And slowly you start to realize that your reflexes are slowing down. You feel as light as a balloon. If you're leafing through a newspaper you'll see that you cannot concentrate on the content of the news, only the headlines. Therefore driving is not recommended after a cycle of chemotherapy.

Next, usually within half an hour, you start to feel nauseous. But not nearly as severe as it's portrayed in films. And many people do not suffer these symptoms. The hospital provides a number of medications (pills to take the day before you start, on the same day, the next day, more or less) that help to alleviate the side effects and make them bearable. Maybe, in my case, it was because I had just been through a pregnancy with constant nausea and vomiting for more than three months, or because I had heard and seen very disturbing things on TV; the truth is that I had prepared for a far more intense sensation than I actually experienced. The effects are rather strong, but they subside after some hours and by the fourth day are barely noticeable, so it's really all about patience, crossing off the days on your calendar and thinking that it's nearly over. Valerian pills are a good help; valerian is a natural sedative herb that calms and helps the time pass.

Ginger infusions are also helpful, which mitigate the nausea, or Coca-Cola; everything is welcome. In the chapter on remedies you will find out how to make marijuana oil, another resource that is quite effective.

From then on, and especially as the cycles occur, you will feel more tired. Sometimes it's hard to leave the house, and indeed some people do not. But I think it is important to set yourself the goal of getting up each morning, taking a shower and even going out to buy bread. During that period I put a little makeup on every day, something that, for me, would have been quite unthinkable until then. The very fact of putting on some eyeliner or a little blusher made me see the day in another light.

Above all, chemo attacks rapidly dividing cells, so you will notice dryness of the mucous membranes, that is, the eyes, nose, vagina and mouth. The chapter given over to remedies offers some basic guidelines to make this period more manageable, although you might not experience this side effect. In fact, I only had canker sores on one occasion. I suppose I later knew how to prevent them. And the genital area dryness I experienced was not painful or too uncomfortable.

However, I did have a lot of concentration difficulties. I would forget my keys, not remember where I left things, or if I had done all errands I had meant to. The good thing about all this is that I could better understand my father, who due to his age had started having lapses of memory. I also felt overwhelmed, unable to make decisions or to plan anything. Deciding what to make for dinner called for a thorough analysis, and recipes that I knew by heart, or intuition, were no longer easy and fun, but challenging. Many women will remember how their memory played tricks on them while they were pregnant. You don't remember who you've explained something to, or where you left your keys. Short-term memory is usually more affected. What you're about to say fades and you seem a little 'detached'. The effect of the chemo I describe causes a similar, more pronounced, effect; fortunately, these are mitigated as the toxins are gradually eliminated from the body.

We discussed all this with the oncologist when I went to have a blood test before the second cycle. He attributed it in part to the lowering of my defences and this was reflected in my blood test. From then on, he prescribed me the famous day-after €1,000 injection, which they give you in the hospital itself (it's not sold in pharmacies). I say famous for several reasons: first is its effectiveness, and second, obviously, for its price, as indeed each jab costs €1,000. Spanish Social Security provides it free of charge (at least when I was being treated), but the price is clearly marked in one corner of the box.

The aim of this injection is to boost the body's defences, stimulating the growth of new and healthy white blood cells. Within 24 to 48 hours after you have undergone chemotherapy you have the jab or inject yourself at home, in the belly, which is a fatty area without muscle. It is a subcutaneous injection, and to administer it you just squeeze the skin between two fingers (as when you pinch your flab) and inject the product, while gradually relaxing the pressure of your hold. We practiced with an orange before my first injection. I suggest you don't read the package leaflet describing the possible side effects of the injection, of which there are many. While I didn't feel any significant differences, we were able to observe that my defences did not drop so much in the subsequent cycles.

The reason that chemotherapy treatment lowers the defences is because, in the same way it destroys tumour cells and cells that reproduce rapidly (such as mucous membranes), it also attacks our antibodies. It is also common to have anemia during treatment for this very reason, since red blood cells are also affected.

The routine procedure for each chemotherapy cycle, if everything goes according to plan – which is what usually happens – is similar. It is defined by days -1 (the day prior to the chemo cycle), 0 (the day of chemo) and day 1 (first day after chemo).

Day -1:
The day before the administration of chemotherapy.
- Early in the morning you have a blood test at the hospital.
- After the analysis, you have an appointment with the oncologist, who assesses the results of the blood test to see whether you are strong enough to undergo another cycle. Sometimes, the doctor may delay treatment to give you more time to recover.
- If the process is to continue, that very night you may have to start taking medication to prevent nausea, muscle aches, heartburn and so forth.

Day 0:
The day you are given chemotherapy.
- In the morning (usually) you go to the hospital to receive treatment.
- Back home, you continue with specific prescribed medication to prevent and mitigate the side effects.
- At night you give yourself the €1,000 injection.

Day 1:
The first day after chemo.
- You probably still have a number of medications to take; it becomes easier every day and decreases as the days pass. Typically, there is up to a three-week period before you begin the process again and tackle the next cycle.

The second half of treatment, when your medication is changed, began, in my case, with the fifth cycle. During the four cycles of chemo that I had left, I was given docetaxel, which acts on the tumour cells that have broken away and spread around the rest of the body.

This treatment is not as directly focused on the tumour as the first. It is responsible for 'cleaning up' malignant cells throughout the body.

I saw out 2009 while receiving my fifth cycle of chemo, the first one with docetaxel. I went to the hospital on December 31st. We had bought some grapes, with which we celebrate the New Year in Spain, just in case I was able to stay awake until midnight and see in the New Year. And yes, we did! This time I didn't get nausea and the first two days were very good. We even had a stroll up in the mountain on January 1st, enjoying glorious sunshine and tranquillity that, in the area, was almost impossible on any other day of the year.

The pain began on the third day. I hadn't been warned about it, I suppose it was to avoid causing undue anxiety. Bone pain is a common side effect with docetaxel. I imagine arthritis causes similar discomfort. And it's unbearable. It feels as though the chest cavity is stretching and shrinking, and your ribs have been subjected to a beating. It lasts several days.

We called the hospital and were recommended alternating paracetamol and ibuprofen every four hours, but it didn't have any effect. So we turned to our neighbourhood pharmacist for help. He recommended muscle relaxants and some kind of natural pills with a relaxing effect, such as valerian, to get me through the rough patch as best as we could. How one appreciates the small gestures of people around you when you feel bad! As we know this pharmacist, we got a painkiller for which you would normally need a prescription. And thank goodness! I think the worst side effect is ignorance, or lack of experience. When the pain first appears and you have not been warned, you don't know where you stand, and this makes everything harder. We didn't know where it was coming from, or how long it would last. We didn't even understand why it occurred. We did notice – especially me, of course – that neither the paracetamol nor the ibuprofen had any effect. So when I saw Joss setting out for the pharmacy, I waited at home wishing with all my might for a solution, but with little confidence. To see him return with the pain relievers was calming in itself. I think the fifth cycle was the worst. In addition to muscle pain,

I had many mouth sores, a fungal infection developed in my mouth and trachea. I could barely eat, and started to salivate uncontrollably. I know of no one who has experienced this sort of salivation. The doctors found it amusing, but it was a drag. I could not relax even ten minutes because my mouth would fill with saliva and I had to spit every now and then. It had also happened when I was pregnant but I managed to control it by chewing gum. Yet the salivation from the chemo was uncontrollable, and with each cycle it became more and more abundant. I will spare you the unpleasant details. I think I have said enough for you to imagine the experience. To give an example, when we were in the car we got used to opening the door so I could spit from time to time, without slowing down too much even if when we were on the motorway. And whenever I left the house I would take a bag filled with paper towels to not spit directly on the ground.

The docetaxel darkened and weakened my nails. I was warned this would happen. They were brittle, and broke off of my fingers. I cut them very short so that they wouldn't get caught on things. And, of course, I painted them a little to disguise them. By now you know me well and so there's no need to add that never before had I taken so much care of them, and so regularly. Until then I painted my nails only for special occasions: weddings, christenings and communions.

And I felt very tired. But I attributed this more to the accumulation of toxins in my body than to the docetaxel itself. I could hardly climb the stairs, because I felt that muscle fatigue you experience when you've been walking all day in the mountains, pushing your body more than it can handle. When I started to notice the pain, I would walk a little more. I don't know whether this was a good idea, but I thought that if every day I went a step further my body would be cleaned of toxins and recover sooner.

I didn't lose much weight, about five kilos. But it showed. Without the wig, I looked like a petrified chicken, my collarbones and ribs protruding and my face pale and downcast. This, of course, I see now in photos. At the time I thought I looked great, with my 'hair' and my 'slim build'.

During treatment some people have diarrhea, and are even admitted to hospital as a precautionary measure to avoid dehydration. Others – I think everyone – retain lots of fluids; although it may not seem so, this is not incompatible with diarrhea. But these are discomforts that happen. Our skin will need to be treated with a special care because it dries out and becomes very sensitive to the sun. It is worth incorporating a total protection sunscreen into our daily hygiene. Chemists' and organic stores sell a number of natural products. We need to prevent the appearance of freckles, blemishes, red and black moles, which don't always disappear with time.

My last cycle of chemotherapy took place on 9th March 2010. Easter week would begin a fortnight later, so we decided to go on holiday to Lisbon to celebrate the end of the process. A friend lent us a beautiful apartment there. It didn't occur to us that Lisbon is a city of hills. On our arrival we found to our surprise that the tram left us in a place from where had to walk about 100 metres downhill to get to the apartment. Once there, we had to climb three floors to the attic! Conclusion: each time we went sightseeing, just getting to the tram involved psyching myself up and a major physical effort. The city is so beautiful and the people so friendly that everything was forgotten when we sat down for a drink or just to take in the scenery from a vantage point.

You feel relieved on the day of the last chemo cycle. You know the worst is over, and henceforth everything will get better. You begin to feel stronger, more alert, more cheerful, and more positive. In a way the threat is now receding. Your skin will recover its suppleness, the bags under your eyes will soften, you'll recover your sense of taste and enjoy meals again, your hair will start to grow. Whether you gained or lost weight, your clothes will look better on you, you'll remember and retain more things and you'll notice how your head and mind respond again. Your day will begin with an extra dose of energy compared to the previous day, and you'll sleep well and soundly. All this makes the side effects of the last cycle seem less severe and not as harsh or as long-lasting.

My mother wanted to spend a few days with me, so she booked a flight for the day after the cycle. I don't know how mothers manage it, but the most surreal things always happen to them. In my case, and on that particular visit, her flight landed in Barcelona on the day of the 'Great Snowfall'. It never snows in Barcelona, and less so in the month of March. Well on that day, 8th March 2010, the snow left the entire city paralyzed. Something that had not happened in fifty years happened on that day. And the situation was even comical. I was at home with a friend who was trying to entertain me, my mother in a taxi that was snowbound in the middle of the road, on her way to my house, and Joss didn't know who to rescue: my mother, from the chaos of Barcelona, or me, from my side effects, the situation – and even my friend, who though trying to help, added some confusion to the scene. It now sounds ridiculous, but it was a storm in a teacup. Add the fact that you have your mother stranded in the middle of a city mired in confusion, with drivers preparing to bed down there and then for the night, and the matter becomes complicated.

Joss was going on a trip for a few days and my mother had come to keep me company and help out. And indeed she helped out more than she could have thought. I plucked up courage, hid my fatigue and put on my best face, welcoming her and making sure she felt comfortable. But for her presence I would have taken longer to bounce back to recovery. Her wish to pamper me and cook me nice little dishes was not so easy to do, not being in her own home with her things around her. So on more than one occasion it was me who ended up cooking for the two of us. It's quite possible that had I been alone, I would have succumbed to my tiredness and eaten less. Having her around, by my side, made the time pass quickly, I was entertained and I think I even felt useful. I didn't want my mother to worry since, in all truth, the situation was not critical, serious, yes, but not critical.

A year and a half has passed since the last cycle of chemotherapy. My feet still feel numb and apparently less flexible, although this is strictly my subjective perception, because reality shows me that I can move as before. When I awake in the morning I feel some pain in my fingers when I move them, as though I had rheumatism or oste-oarthritis. My fingertips also retain a tingling reminder and the loss of sensitivity I had at the time. You do not entirely lose your sense of touch. Rather, some fingers feel as if the skin were a little rougher and thus unable to recall the information they once had, like when you stick a piece of cellophane on your fingertip and notice a strange sensation. They are mere recollections of those effects, already a distant memory. I think they will gradually disappear. They say it takes up to two years to eliminate the toxins. I have a lifetime to observe how these effects abate.

I don't regret having gone through the chemotherapy. I sometimes think it's not so important what you do but how you do it. Chemotherapy is one way to treat a tumour and eliminate it. If you believe in it, go ahead, because that will give you strength to overcome the tumour from inside yourself, too, from within. So long as you make an informed decision about what you are doing and are aware of why you are doing it.

It's very easy to say that the chemo is poison. In fact, I think so myself, because it really has an impact on the body with extremely unpleasant ramifications. But even so, I also believe in the body's ability to regenerate, to find its equilibrium and forge ahead, whatever we do. We mistreat our body so much and so often!

Not only with medications, but also with what we eat, what we drink, the pace of life we lead, the sleepless hours, the rush, worries, too much sun, exercise, or sedentary living, fashionable high heels, bad postures, computers, radiation, and so forth. Even so, our body continues to give us its all, and resist. So, if the reason for not having chemo is the fear of the side effects involved, there are ways to help our body recover and to alleviate the severity of the experience. Hence the importance of nutrition and complementary or alternative therapies, such as Chinese medicine, which helped me heal my liver and kidney from the first day, or homotoxicology, which I began at the end of the chemotherapy.

Surgery

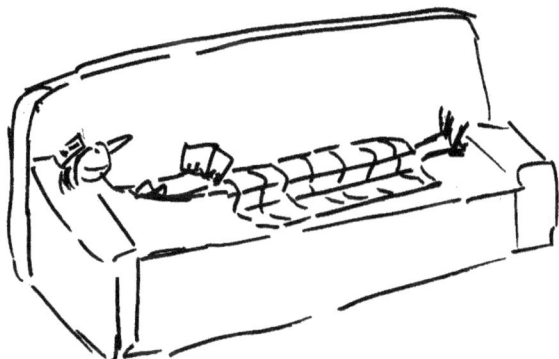

Having an operation is always an assault on the body. And yet, I think that breast cancer surgery is much more bearable than it might seem. There is no reason to feel scared. Surgeons perform several every day.

In the Western world we don't attach much importance to going into an operating theatre. It seems almost a formality. TCM, however, views surgery as a highly invasive technique, which causes considerable damage and an energy imbalance. Gradually, operations undermine our body's vital energy. According to TCM, we are all born with a specific amount of life force. It is our energy 'pool', which we consume by living life, and it cannot be replenished. Attacks such as surgery consume the extra energy needed to recover, which depletes our reserves.

Things to consider

Breast surgery, especially if it involves the removal of the lymph nodes, involves a long recovery process. There are two stages to get through, for which we can prepare psychologically, and also from an organizational standpoint.

The first stage begins as soon as you are discharged from hospital and get home. You will have little mobility, and you'll ache, so it's best to plan in advance the needs you may have, so as not to have to resort to improvised solutions on the days following the operation. I mean simple things like having meals ready, having comfortable underwear, accepting the fact your arm will be immobilized, and although we feel more or less well, we cannot carry loads, cook, make the bed, go shopping or dress the children.

The second stage is lengthier and harder. It takes months to regain full mobility, and to achieve this you need to be unswerving. The secret – which is not really a secret at all – is to move the arm as much as possible, stretch it, and prevent the scar tissue from forming.

Do not let the arm become resigned to stiffness. It is not difficult to regain full mobility, but you must have the right frame of mind. You are embarking on an exceptional period during which your body is working to heal itself, and it needs some extra doses of love, time and effort. The doctor or hospital physical therapist will usually show you the right exercises to do on a daily basis. And these are the key to recovery, even though they will hurt a little. The pain will ease with time, although it seems impossible, and you will gradually be able to raise your arm higher and stretch further without problems.

Surgery and its side effects

You are normally admitted to hospital the night before the surgery, or on that same morning if you are scheduled to have the operation in the afternoon. The operation itself is very quick. It usually lasts no more than two hours.

When I went in on a Thursday around four in the afternoon, I was put in a room with another patient and her family. She didn't speak much, nor could she. She was surrounded by people and commotion! Between the ubiquitous TV (an accident and crime programme, to be exact) that was on full blast and that no one was watching, her teenage daughter on her mobile phone, the daughter's friend, and all the relatives, including a man who was asleep on the couch with his feet on the bed and his shirt unbuttoned, I found myself in a truly Dantesque setting. All I wanted was some peace and quiet! Some ten different people were constantly coming and going, with bags of crisps and more than a few comments. The highlight came when the poor woman felt sick (no wonder, I suppose she needed some air) and went to the bathroom for a moment. The family, rather than go out and leave her alone, followed her into the bathroom!

It was surreal, I remember affectionately, because she turned out to be a really lovely woman. She turned off the TV, got her family to leave, and by the next day had been discharged, leaving me alone in the room.

The next morning went fast. Shortly after I woke up I was given a tranquilizer (another protocol – they say the anesthesia works best this way) and was taken through the hospital in a wheelchair to have a couple of tests. I was a bit 'high', somewhat tipsy, and in excellent spirits.

Of the operating theatre I can say little because they put you out straight away. But the journey back to the room was tremendous. I was half awake, but felt like I was on a cloud. Anesthesia leaves you stupidly happy. I had an IV in my left arm, connected to saline and medications, and my entire chest at the height of my breast was wrapped in a hard, white and tight bandage, which also served as a corset. A tube had been inserted into my right side, under the armpit, where I had had surgery, which was connected to a plastic bottle. Known as a Redon drain, this is a bottle that collects lymph fluid drained as a result of lymph node manipulation during surgery. Each day the amount collected is recorded, until hardly any more fluid is produced because the body has found alternative drainage pathways. Then (usually between five and ten days after the operation) it is removed.

I was brought back to my room from the operating theatre and put back into bed. As my roommate had vacated the bed next to the window, we had the idea of moving there to enjoy the light. Joss took care of this. I just listened with a look of joy of on my face, extremely grateful for everyone being so nice. And straight after suggesting my moving to the window, they began to push my bed on wheels together with all the tubes connected to me (because instead of moving you, they move the whole bed with you in it, something that hadn't occurred to me, of course). The manoeuvre seemed so complicated that I suddenly said, "Wait, I'll help." And I almost got up! They found it so hilarious that they roared with laughter, and I did not understand anything. My offer seemed so natural to me, but now I understand. And imagining the scene makes me smile. I was not even able to move. With all the tubes hanging off of me and the operation so recent, how could I even contemplate the possibility of getting out of bed? Moreover pushing the bed myself, as though I were as fresh as a daisy. The anesthesia gave me such a feeling of bliss and well-being that I believed I was capable of anything when, in all honesty, I couldn't have even lifted a finger!

The day after the operation the corset was removed and my wounds were cleaned. The surgeons had used the same butterfly clips that had been used to close the portacath incision.

I was discharged on Sunday. I went home with a drain connected and hanging from the wound under my arm and wrapped in a bag. Every three days I returned to the hospital to have the dressing changed and follow-up. They measured the fluid in the Redon bottle and made sure that everything was going according to plan.

After the operation, I was concerned about not being able to move my arm. So I started to exercise from day one. Some people don't recover all their mobility, especially because they decide not to move their arm while the wound still hurts, should it open up. Although it's hard to believe, after the incision has been closed, it is really difficult to open as long as your movements are gentle. Therefore, it is best to stretch your arm every day, forcing it up a bit more, but not sharply. This is the only way to make a complete recovery.

Regarding scar tissue, there are also ways to help soften and heal it. The chapter on remedies includes some guidelines on how to do this.

Radiotherapy

It is an entirely different treatment from chemotherapy. It involves exposing the tumour area to beams of radiation, with the intention of destroying any malignant cells that might have remained. The radiation is intelligent, in that it knows how to discriminate between cells, and directly focuses on potentially cancerous cells, but the fact is that some healthy tissue is damaged. Radiotherapy sessions are carried out daily. I had thirty-three sessions. They last no longer than five minutes, including the time it takes to undress and put you in the right position. Its brevity does not mean the radiation dose is harmless. It is an aggressive treatment. For some people it causes fatigue, but I think this is largely due to the effort of having to travel to the hospital every day.

Things to consider

It's hugely important to prepare your skin before starting radiotherapy; I would almost say this is the most important part, because for more than a month you will be subjected to a daily assault that, though neither painful or noticeable, leaves its mark.

Pharmacies and hospitals usually recommend using pharmaceutical creams developed specifically for the period of radiation therapy, twice daily. I chose to avoid chemicals. Having studied the properties of the active ingredients in these creams, I decided to create a natural alternative that provides similar benefits.

The pharmaceutical cream that I took as a starting point to develop my own cream contained urea and vitamin E. I was not tempted by the option of using urea itself, a compound found in our urine, so I replaced it with another product with the same properties. I was mainly looking to reproduce its ability to retain the skin's natural moisture. Vitamin E is a regenerator and antioxidant. My homemade remedy was as follows:

❖ *Wheat germ oil:* It is the most abundant source of vitamin E that exists in nature. It has regenerative and antioxidant effects and is very moisturizing and nourishing.

❖ *Aloe vera:* As a substitute for urea. One of its major properties is that it is an excellent moisturizer. It is also a powerful bactericide and has potent cell regeneration properties, favouring the healing of injuries. It is available as a gel and when applied to the skin produces a cooling effect.

Both products can be easily found at herbalist shops and natural food stores.

Two weeks before beginning radiotherapy I started applying the treatment. Several times a day I mixed the two products in my hand and applied them generously over the area that was to be radiated. I applied it so thickly that the oils impregnated my underwear and sheets. I bought cotton bras without underwire that I had to restock often, that's true, but it was worth it. My radiologist was so amazed with the results that she asked me for my remedy, because the radiation barely burnt the skin tissue. Plus, I have very sensitive skin. It gets covered in spots when exposed to the sun, and burns easily. Now, one year on, there are no differences between the irradiated skin and the skin that wasn't; irradiated areas usually acquire a darker tone.

Radiotherapy treatment and its side effects

The truth is that thanks to all the precautions I took, I hardly noticed the radiotherapy. It was very tolerable. Physically, it wasn't a problem. On April 9th I underwent surgery. The healing of the wound and post-operative treatment lasted until early May. My radiotherapy sessions began on the 28th of that month. Six weeks had elapsed since the last session of chemo. I was starting to regain my strength and was feeling well. I was still somewhat tired, but saw so many 'green shoots' that encouraged me, so many positive changes in my body making every day better than the last, that the radiotherapy seemed like just another treatment. The truth is that I had it pretty easy. It took less than ten minutes to go by scooter from home to the hospital, ten to fifteen in the waiting room, then the session itself, and back home. In an hour or so I was done. And everything you hear about you losing your appetite, or feeling tired or not wanting to do anything – I didn't notice. Perhaps people who have to travel many miles to get to the hospital experience it differently, or those who do suffer burns, but I experienced nothing of the sort. The treatment seemed long but it was bearable. That said, it would be a mistake to think that radiotherapy is a mild or superficial treatment. Whereas the effects of chemo are felt at the time, some side effects to radiotherapy can take years to appear, and they are irreversible. Aside from burns and skin ulcers, which are quite frequent, the irradiated skin may acquire a colour darker than the rest of the skin, and this effect is permanent. Some people get very tired, and this fatigue may last for months. Others suffer burns to internal organs such as the lungs, which cause a drop in respiratory capacity, and a dry cough may develop that can become chronic.

Furthermore, radiotherapy often affects the lymph nodes and promotes the development of lymphedema. It can also burn certain nerve endings (which are rare in the case of a breast tumour, since the area exposed to radiation does not have nerves) which, with the passing of time, can mean loss of mobility. I would never think of downplaying this treatment.

Tamoxifen

After chemotherapy, and if the tumour is not hormone dependent (see 'Types and phases of tumours'), the 'breast cancer treatment' continues with the ingestion of a daily pill, for five years, whose active ingredient is tamoxifen. Doctors offer tamoxifen as the magic pill that inhibits the estrogen production. If the tumour is hormone dependent, and therefore sensitive to estrogen, medical reasoning asserts that by artificially eliminating the production of estrogen in our bodies, which is the tumour's power supply, we will decrease the chances of developing a tumour in the breast. Therefore, tamoxifen is proposed as a solution to block the production of the 'food' the tumour needs to appear and develop.

At this point, I do not know if it is necessary to clarify that I chose not to take it. And I'm very pleased with my decision.

For several reasons: the first and foremost is that I find it hard to believe that tamoxifen has more advantages than disadvantages. I think tumours occur for other reasons, and that's what one has to focus on. I find it quite unnatural to prevent the body from producing the hormones it needs to prevent the proliferation of a tumour that, from the outset, we are not certain will reappear. In addition, tamoxifen is no guarantee that you will not relapse. It simply reduces risk percentages.

Things to consider

Tamoxifen has certain implications that are important to know before jumping blindly into treatment. The first is that for the two to five-year duration of the treatment, you cannot have children. If we add another year to detoxify the body before attempting pregnancy, the time period is significant. The second involves all the side effects it causes, and with which you have to live during the process. These are effects that, in many cases, the doctors still do not know themselves. The third factor to bear in mind is that you continue supplying the body with chemicals that go against its nature.

Tamoxifen and its side effects

My oncologist knew from the start that I would not want to take it. As we progressed with chemotherapy, we both gradually developed a good rapport. He saw that I pondered every step I took and that I questioned him about them. He saw my position regarding the tumour and life itself: he saw it coming. In addition, certain situations he had witnessed during his practice made him more permeable to the subject of motherhood. He did his job flawlessly. At the end of chemo, when the time came to suggest the option of tamoxifen, he had done his homework. Using a computer programme my oncologist had calculated, based on statistics, the odds of having both a relapse and dying in the next ten years. These probabilities analyzed the following parameters:

❖ Only undergo surgery
❖ Undergo surgery and chemotherapy
❖ Undergo surgery and take tamoxifen

To my complete surprise, tamoxifen 'guaranteed' me a 6% greater likelihood of survival. We were already working in a roughly 90% chance after everything I had done. And the statistical programme did not include radiation therapy, which certainly adds 5%.

That is how I made my choice about tamoxifen. And thus I decided not to take it. It wasn't worth it. I had the support and tranquillity of all the alternative therapies I was following, which marked an important aid in my recovery.

Of course, each woman is free to make her own choice; what's more, we all have the responsibility to do so. The numbers, the statistics – even the experiences that others may share with you – do not contribute much. I saw my decision very clearly because it is what I feel, what my body asked me to do. It is not so much the desire to have children as the desire to let my body find its balance, giving it what I believe helps it naturally, always rowing with the current, rather than acting by modifying natural biological processes.

When we stop producing estrogen a series of changes take place in our body that will generate several side effects, in many cases similar to those of menopause (hot flushes, vaginal dryness, irregular periods, etc.).

Tamoxifen causes a wide range of side effects.

❖ First, it can bring on thrombosis, i.e. blood clots in the veins, which can cause blockages with varying risks. This is one of the causes of myocardial infarction.
❖ It also increases the chances of developing uterine cancer.
❖ It may also cause excessive fatigue, concentration problems, fainting, light-headedness, etc.
❖ In some cases it may give rise to an intolerance that generates joint problems, swelling, pain, etc.
❖ Moreover, tamoxifen is incompatible with pregnancy.

I know several women who have taken it. All of them have described some of the side effects mentioned in the list, and were so intense that in some cases they had to halt the treatment. One of these women has symptoms of depression because her desire to be a mother has been shattered by the tamoxifen.

Many of these side effects are not even documented and come as a surprise to the clinicians. I speak of what I have seen in close acquaintances, cases of friends, etc. I dare not imagine what may be happening to other people who I don't even know.

There are still many knowledge gaps in the field of hormone therapy and its correlation with tumours. Different doctors advocate contradictory positions. Some will prescribe tamoxifen for five years to inhibit hormone production, and others will encourage you to get pregnant as a natural antidote to the recurrences. Therefore, Western medicine does not have all the answers, and I think that sometimes it's better not to act and instead give nature a chance to find its own solutions before resorting to chemical and external solutions. This may require some time and trust.

In the next chapter we will look at some alternatives.

Chapter Five

ALTERNATIVE AND COMPLEMENTARY MEDICINES AND THERAPIES

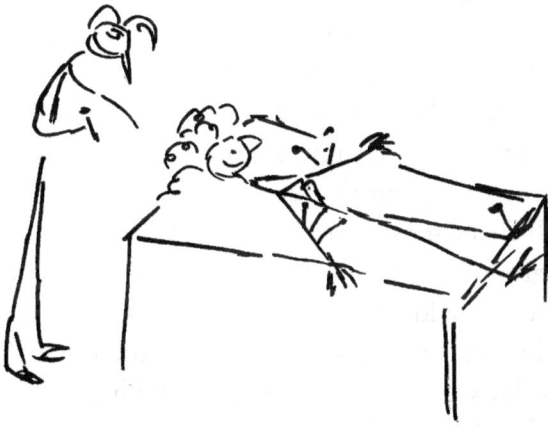

Curative Therapies

Traditional Chinese Medicine

Just as I have not passed judgement on other treatments or classified them as good or bad, here I will likewise just mention the experience I had as a beneficiary of TCM, and share some of the information I have. It's hard to be neutral when something works well for one, and my experience with TCM has not only helped me restore my health, but has also opened a new path of exploration and experimentation in all fields of life.

When my lump was discovered in August 2009, I had the good fortune to find a Chinese master whom I began to visit before starting conventional treatment. I recall how, after having asked me a few general questions and then examined my tongue, hand and eyes, he made me lie down on an examination table and remained silent, sensing, thinking. His treatment to solve the problem consisted of, from the first visit, placing herbs, roots and some acupuncture needles in different parts of my body. During the year I was his patient, his working tools were phytotherapy (the use of medicinal plants and herbs), acupuncture (the use of very fine needles to alter the energy of the body), and to a lesser extent, diet. Depending on how he saw me he would sometimes change the point where he inserted the needle. If I had nausea he focused on decreasing its effect; if I was tired he helped me regain my energy. All this while he worked to rebalance my energy and to prevent the tumour from reappearing.[11]

Master Jin's diagnosis was a breath of fresh air at a time when everything around me weighed me down. First he said, "Don't fret." He continued by adding that I indeed had a malignant tumour to deal with, but that the first organ to be cured was the brain (Jin called it my 'boss'). Imagine my surprise. We had just met, and with his half-broken Spanish I first assumed I had brain cancer! I finally understood what he was saying. My problem had originated in the brain, because my 'boss' had suffered an imbalance and sent the wrong orders to the rest of my body. He told me that this imbalance had particularly manifested itself in my breast. According to Master Jin, the healing process would begin by healing the 'boss', from where we would check the growth of the tumour and shrink it.

He told me, "You, before, angry many years, right?". How could I deny it. It was not exactly anger, but I had experienced some years of

---

11. We saw in chapter 1 that TCM views a tumour as the body's response to an energy imbalance. In order to heal a tumour at its root, it's necessary to recover our energy balance.

searching that made me unhappy with myself, and lacking in self-esteem. I was doing piecework, not considering my own needs.

I wasn't giving myself the same love I gave to others, and I forgot to take care of myself. He saw it clearly. His acute perception, knowledge of a culture and codes that are still beyond our comprehension, enabled him to read me with extraordinary ease, simply from my level of energy, to which he gained access merely by looking at me. In this case, he was able to perceive everything because my liver was sending signs of deterioration and imbalance. TCM explains how the liver is extremely sensitive to our emotions. It suffers when we experience stress, anger or rage, which ultimately leads to a malfunctioning of the body itself. This explains why, in the long run, what begins as a simple energy imbalance brought on by emotional causes can lead to more serious illnesses.

This great master was also the first to establish a link between my tumour, my mood and other imbalances in my body (my thyroid gland dysfunction, the uterine fibroids). Doctors of Western medicine never established such relationships despite my insistent questions. And this is the huge difference between the medicines known as integral, or holistic, and Western medicine. Integrative medicine sees the human being as a whole, in which all the dysfunctions of the body provide clues about what may be happening. Western medicine by contrast focuses and acts on each of the clues separately, without linking them to others, unless they are obvious.

What I have explained is my understanding of Master Jin's diagnosis, although I am aware that I fail to understand the essence of the medicine he practises. TCM uses codes that differ greatly from ours. It is not only the language; what sets it apart is the culture, the priorities, a way of understanding the world, the planet and its interrelationship with us. It is even a way of understanding life. The great fortune we have is that TCM works; there is no need to understand it. Just go to a good professional.

After that first appointment with Master Jin, I almost floated out of his office. He continued to treat me for months. Throughout the process he was with me every step of the way, sharing in silence my fears, my weaknesses and infirmities, my side effects. And every day his maxim was: "Don't fret" and "Every day you're stronger. Your energy is very good. "

I noticed that the state of happiness that came over me after acupuncture was not happenstance, and not only brought on by the words he uttered. It went deeper, was able to have an impact on my emotions, and fine-tune my energy. What seemed ominous and shocking before lying down on his examination table, he managed to turn into a situation that I had to go through, and which I was able to face with strength and optimism.

Master Jin has been able to make me a much happier person, more in touch with myself, more secure and confident, and much stronger. We have never exchanged words. I don't think it is necessary. By merely observing me, he perceives my energy and this conveys much more than all the words in the world. From this experience, I have reached two critical conclusions:

> ➤ The first is that there is *no magic formula that will materialize from the outside and solve our problems*, whether it be a tumour, a depression or a bankruptcy. Miracles occur from within us, we are the key to making change happen.

> ➤ The second conclusion is that *whatever you do, it is essential to trust it, you must believe in it, even if you don't understand it.* An acupuncture needle will achieve nothing if you do not play your part, neither will the strongest chemotherapy. Our brain is so strong that it can block the development of the disease, or the effects of medication. Therefore it is very important that our minds and our actions work in conjunction, taking the same direction. Because the best way to ensure a successful outcome to the treatment we choose is to give it everything we can, both pure action and the energy of our thoughts.

Homotoxicology

Not all alternative therapies are millennia-old sciences. There is a new way of understanding medicine, somewhere between Western medicine and homeopathy, called homotoxicology. It is a school that uses the latest generation of natural medications that provide the body with what it needs to heal.

TCM focuses on the individual as a whole, while homotoxicology, like Western medicine, studies cells to understand what is happening.

From there, it seeks ways to modify the behaviour of these malignant cells and to cleanse the body. This approach involves working with synthesized plant extracts, powerful antioxidants, and other natural principles that are administered to the patient. According to homotoxicology, diseases occur primarily because the patient's cells are suffering a high level of toxicity (this may be caused by a lack of oxygen, excess acidity in the blood, and so on). The patient alone is unable to eliminate these toxins, which accumulate and eventually manifest themselves as disease. Sometimes our body is unable to produce certain substances that would help to remove these toxins, and that is when homotoxicology supplies them through an external approach. Thus homotoxicology detoxifies our bodies at the cellular level, strengthens our immune system and restores our body with everything it needs to cure itself. So our body is responsible for the healing.

There is documented data confirming spectacular healings. People with metastases in the brain, with different types of cancer or other conditions have recovered their health. There is ever-growing support for this non-invasive medicine, which has no side effects and works. Many oncologists and specialists in different fields of medicine are beginning to learn about it and utilize this new medical approach.

I discovered homotoxicology when I finished the chemotherapy. I had just had surgery, and already felt strong enough to start something new. At first I believed that homotoxicology only served to clean the chemical residues from previous conventional treatments, and would help me recover faster. Now I realized that my vision of it was limited. After my first interview with the doctor I understood its scope and enormous potential. Homotoxicology is really an alternative to chemotherapy, and to radiotherapy. I chose to combine all treatments. Homotoxicology gave me the certainty that I was harnessing everything in my power to help my body to regain its health – not only the strength that I had lost as a result of chemotherapy and radiotherapy, but the balance I was lacking and which had resulted in the appearance of the tumour. In addition to TCM, I embarked on a new path in search of healing. A natural path focusing, once again, on the root of the problem, and I approached it as such, using the knowledge that science has developed to date. The way to address this was still finding the body's natural balance to restore it to health, only this time reflected at a cellular level.

The homotoxicologist carried out several tests on me. Using electrodes, he listened to the responses in my gut to check their state. He also examined my iris, skin, tongue, and my whole body. He felt my tummy and, as Master Jin did, told me that my tumour had originated in the uterus, although the problematic cells had not been strong enough to spread. One of them, taking advantage of a moment of weakness, when my body was not on its guard and my defences unable to neutralize it (does it or does it not make sense to believe that the impact of my pregnancy and the loss of my baby was the a cause of my lump?), had settled in my breast, where it was able to grow.

Both doctors insisted on the importance of the interrelationship of the thyroid, breast and uterus. Unlike my oncologist, who never attached importance to my hypothyroidism (a malfunction of the thyroid gland) or the fibroids on my ovaries (small benign cysts), both Master Jin and the homotoxicologist considered these as fundamental, and devoted much energy to cleansing the thyroid.

It's hard to describe homotoxicological treatment because like TCM, which works primarily with acupuncture and herbal medicine (herbs, plants and roots), homotoxicology utilizes many types and formats of products. In fact, I know several people who have visited my doctor for a lump in their breast and the treatments they were prescribed were all very different. They tend to last for several months, during which the patient consumes large amounts of natural products, nutritional supplements, homeopathic supplements, and during this time he or she also receives weekly injections of substances that their body needs, as well as vitamin C, a powerful antioxidant and regenerator that helps healthy cells to multiply in order to heal the body quickly. All this moreover strengthens the immune system.

Homotoxicology is a non-invasive Western approach, based on scientific research, and supported by documented findings on patients. It is still relatively unknown because it is a new approach, but everything suggests that it will become an ever increasing method for acting on and attacking illnesses.

Supportive therapies

In addition to the main therapeutic options, such as TCM and homotoxicology, which in themselves offer alternatives to conventional treatments, there are other therapies that help to maximize the effects of chemotherapy, for example, and alleviate the side effects caused by it.

Ozonotherapy

Ozone therapy uses medical grade ozone as a working tool. Ozone is a variety of oxygen which is formed in the upper layers of the atmosphere. The type used for therapeutic purposes is not pure ozone, but a combination of this and oxygen that is applied in doses that are decided depending on the type of treatment. It is called medical grade ozone.

The emergence and development of tumour cells is associated with a lack of oxygen in the body. One of the best ways to fight them is to create an oxygenated environment in which they cannot live or reproduce.

Noteworthy among the properties of ozone is its oxygenating capacity. By supplying ozone to our body, our blood is able to absorb more oxygen, which better transports this to our cells. As a result of its application, it creates an environment in our body in which it is more difficult for cancer cells to reproduce and survive. Moreover, when the body receives blood that is more oxygenated, it works better. That is, our cells better transport the nutrients they need and are able to do their work more easily. This enhanced performance allows for faster recovery from fatigue or diseases, since it facilitates the regeneration of body tissues, enhances our immunological capacity and also increases the body's ability to produce natural anti-inflammatories. Therefore, by using a natural and harmless a medium such as ozone, we are helping our body to work better.

Another outstanding property of medical grade ozone is its anti-oxidant effect. It is an effective tool for counteracting oxidative stress generated by multiple causes such as anxiety, poor eating habits, radiation, etc. Oxidative stress occurs when our body is unable to rid itself of all the oxidant toxins it generates. Their presence in the body is directly related to aging and diseases like diabetes, cancer and Alzheimer's.

Let us recall what was said by Still, the father of osteopathy, who we mentioned in Chapter 2: "the brain is the best pharmacy in the world". Therefore, if we facilitate the flow of blood throughout our body, and if that blood is more oxygenated, we will stimulate our large pharmacy, which will send the best solution to every place in our body.

Hence, ozone therapy enhances the effect of chemotherapy on the tumour being treated, because both external medication and our own natural defences and healing tools will better reach the affected area. Ozone multiplies the effectiveness of conventional treatments, and it also makes us feel better, thanks to the revitalizing effect it provides.

There are several ways to administer ozone. One is by the so-called 'autosanguis' therapy. The doctor performing the treatment first extracts some blood. Then, a machine combines it with ozone. The next step is to re-inject this blood back into your body, once treated. Absorption is immediate.

In my case, both the therapist and I agreed that I had already received too many injections from the other treatments. Between the blood tests, the chemo, the injection given beforehand to prevent my defences from lowering, and I don't know how many others, not one week had gone by without having something injected into me. So we opted for an alternative option, which is the administration of ozone through the rectum.

I went twice a week to the doctor's practice and in ten minutes I was done. It's a strange feeling, which one is usually hesitant to discuss. A cannula is used to deliver the ozone through the anus into the intestines. It doesn't hurt, it's simply different. Sometimes it gives one the immediate urge to go to the bathroom. And if so, nothing happens, no effect is lost nor is any ozone expelled, as our rectum absorbs at the same rate we breathe.

Whether it's thanks to the ozone, TCM, or both, my oncologist was amazed how much my tumour had shrunk since starting chemo. Given that it was unaggressive and slow growing, a slow or insignificant reduction was expected. It actually shrunk by almost 90%; something that had surpassed the calculations and predictions made.

Neural therapy

Neural therapy is used to treat scars, to help re-establish nerve endings between the tissues cut by an incision, caused by either a deep wound or surgery.

When our skin has a wound, or an open operation is performed, the incision in the skin removes with it veins, capillaries, as well as nerves. Many of our tissues regenerate quickly and the wound gradually closes up. But the skin never entirely heals. Scar tissue is different, less flexible and more sensitive (so scars must always be protected from burns, and moisturized more than the rest of the skin, especially while still fresh).

Aside from the regeneration of skin tissue that on the surface can be seen with the naked eye, there are other tissues that do not regenerate so quickly. Everyone has probably felt at one time numbness or a lack of feeling in the tissue surrounding a wound. This is the result of cut nerve endings that are unable to transmit what they perceive. Unfortunately, the capacity to regenerate nerve endings is not as great as that of other tissues. Over time, some feeling may be regained, but it is a long process.

Neural therapy is a treatment that acts directly on the scars. It involves the use of a compound called procaine, which is directly injected in small amounts into many points along the line of the scar. Procaine is made in a laboratory and is mainly used as an anesthetic, but in neural therapy it is used for its ability to create 'bridges' between nerve endings. That is, when a nerve has been cut, procaine can be used to re-establish 'bridges' between the cut endings, so that they may once again transmit information. Procaine does not regenerate tissue, but creates a new communication channel linking the two separated endings so that impulses may flow again.

I was late in discovering this therapy, and I find it surprising that nothing is said about it, even in hospitals. Something as simple as treating my scar by injecting it once with an anesthetic has helped me regain some feeling in my underarm and upper arm. It can be used on all types of scars and, from my point of view, it's highly recommended.

Body movement therapy

Thus far we have mainly spoken of largely static therapies in which the patient 'allow themselves to be treated,' participating with their discipline, their strength and their good will towards the treatment, being aware of the importance of believing in themselves and in what is being done to them for the therapy to work.

However, for our entire body to function it is also essential to be active. And it is in our power to achieve this. Anything that involves keeping our body in motion is welcome. Going out, having a stroll, interacting with others, is important.

Walking

During my treatment, we would often spend weekends in the mountains. It was winter – ski season – but I found it too arduous to carry the equipment, don those heavy clothes, and so forth. So we eventually established a routine, which consisted of Joss going skiing in the morning while I stayed home working on a puzzle, meditating, reading a book, or simply doing nothing. When Joss finished he would call me, and I would leave the house where we were staying and walk down the road where he would be coming from. Normally we would meet up after forty minutes or an hour. I'd walk about four kilometres downhill. Knowing that he was coming to meet me and that I wouldn't have to reserve my strength to walk back made the stroll much more enjoyable.

The contact with nature charged up my batteries and back at the house, conscious that I'd had a good stroll, I felt enormously gratified because although I felt tired, I was proving to myself that I was still very active, enjoying the little things in life, and that my body was responding. It is therefore very important to keep moving, no matter how tired you feel.

Water Sports

Some people enjoy practising water aerobics because it facilitates very effortless movements. Essentially it is aerobic exercises done in a pool,

125

to the rhythm of music. Swimming is also a good choice to stimulate and awaken the body, without being exhausting.

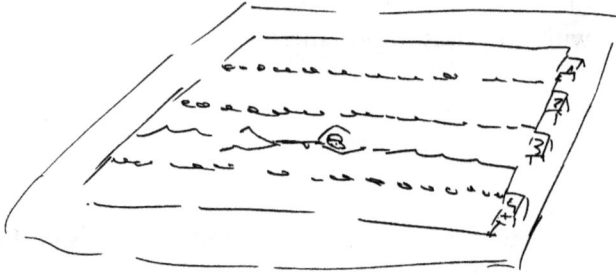

Oriental Disciplines

Yoga is also an excellent tool. It is a discipline of physical and mental work. It mobilizes energy and gives you peace and balance. There are many types of yoga, and sometimes it is not easy to choose between one and the other. My proposal is, regardless of what it's called (kundalini yoga, integral yoga, Sivananda yoga, hatha yoga, ten-tchi yoga, dynamic yoga, vinyasa yoga), look for a type in which you can perform gentle exercises, breathing techniques and meditation. In our situation it is not necessary to adopt overly complicated postures or maintain them for long. Instead, it is important to calm your mind, and breathing and meditation are essential to achieve this. Positive visualization will help us to feel closer to the end, to enjoy the process a little bit and to keep in mind that its end is your full recovery.

Within the group of Oriental techniques there are more options. One is *Qigong*. It is a practice that has been used in China for thousands of years to maintain and improve health. It is intimately linked to TCM, which considers Qigong as one of its fundamental preventive treatments. Through a series of exercises, or static postures, you work your life force, strengthening and balancing it, and undoing blockages, and so forth.

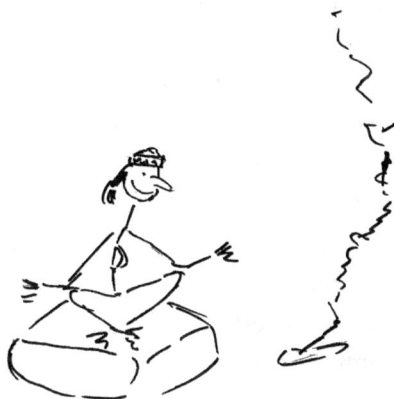

T'ai chi ch'uan is a gentle Chinese martial art that seeks peace and balance through relaxed and harmonious exercises.

Posturology

A couple of months before I knew I would have a difficult year as a result of the breast tumour, I had reached an agreement with an amazing woman to acquaint companies with posturology, also called global postural recalibration.

Alicia is the director of the health centre I attended to practise different kinds of body work, ranging from yoga to African dance, Pilates and posturology.

One day during the summer, between classes, I was chatting with a small group of students while we were doing some stretching exercises. Alicia was there, taking part in the conversation and helping us with the exercises. For some reason, the conversation turned to Alicia's work, and her desire to acquaint companies with what she was doing at her centre. I thought it was an excellent idea. I saw there was much potential in her work, and a great need to bring body awareness to the business world. So right there and then we decided to put into practice the idea, and began to work together on a new project aimed at promoting an interest in the body as an integral and fundamental part of the individual, in training schools, companies and business groups.

This book has shown us, in many ways and through different approaches, that everything passes through the body: emotions, stress, worries, and life experiences. Posturology, applies and moves beyond this premise. It provides us with tools to learn how to manage our health. The discipline begins with a knowledge of one's body. Therefore all posturology classes include detailed explanations of what you are doing at each moment. Once we know our body, we begin to understand it. From there, and through specific, highly varied exercises (some centered on physical movement, some on energy, others on osteopathic techniques), our goal is to recognize what happens in our bodies and act on the cause of the problem, in order to find balance. Posturology is a therapy aimed at caring for our body without resorting to external solutions, whether drugs, operations or prostheses. The key to solving a physical problem is to understand what is happening. From there on, we focus on recovering our freedom of movement, and on every part of our body regaining its space and natural rhythm. The ultimate goal of posturology is to make each one of us responsible for our health.

Two weeks after my meeting with Alicia I went to see her again with my diagnosis. My idea was to defer our joint venture. I didn't know what to expect once I started chemotherapy, and I didn't think I could give my best under the effects of the drugs. To launch a new project requires, in addition to enthusiasm and confidence, unflagging energy, which I might not have in the months that lay ahead of me.

But Alicia was able to see beyond this. She is a respectful person but doesn't shy from giving her opinion. She speaks to you gently and affectionately, so you can decide with all the information at hand. She spoke about Hamer, gave me Master Jin's phone number, and helped me to view my tumour in a different light. So thanks to the tumour, I was able to find holistic medical therapists that I had been looking for so many years, and make contact with a group of people who lived by its precepts. Surely, had she been in my place, Alicia would have opted for a different treatment than the one I chose, but my arguments helped her understand my reasons.

During the months following that first conversation, far from putting aside our idea, Alicia and I worked together, went out to dinner, laughed, cried, and supported one another and gradually explored a beautiful project.

Unexpectedly, posturology became part of my life. I was suddenly immersed in a new world that opened its doors to me. On the one hand, I absorbed its methodology, during long conversations with Alicia that eventually became articles or content for our website. And on the other, I put into practice everything I learned when I went to class, or in my daily life, in my meditations, in my relationship with myself and with others.

They say that nothing happens by chance. When you are searching for something you end up getting answers to your questions, and it happened in this case. I found it in posturology and in Alicia, and our paths proved to converge.

We left our heavy loads at the door and offered each other our personal gifts to continue to improve ourselves together. My process and outcome since the emergence of the tumour would not have been the same but for this encounter, because in classes, talks and visits to the centre I recharged my batteries and consolidated myself in this view of life. We are responsible for ourselves and our disease, and also for our enormous capacity to achieve what we set out to do, because the secret is always within us.

Other therapies

There are many other therapies that can help us. Below I explain a few that I have not tried personally. Like those mentioned above, they are tools we can utilize in difficult times like these. They can provide tranquillity and calmness in the face of anxiety and weariness caused by the situation. They can further our healing process and help in daily life.

Biomagnetism

Like TCM, this therapy holds that the body is healthy and in balance when energy flows through it normally. Disease takes hold when certain points are altered.

Once a diagnosis and study have been carried out to identify the parts of our body that have experienced a distortion, the therapy itself involves applying magnets to specific points on the body to rebalance it. By changing our energy field we also modify our pH. Biomagnetism attempts to re-establish the body's alkaline pH, in which tumour cells do not survive, and so the disease disappears.

Shiatsu

Shiatsu is a traditional Japanese therapy that treats the body through its energy pathways, and incorporates concepts of TCM into its knowledge base. The therapist applies pressure to specific points of the body, with the intention to clear energy blockages. By unblocking our meridians and reopening our channels, energy flows, which ensures our body's balance and health. Shiatsu works on those areas of the body used in acupuncture, and incorporates body movements and stretching that allow access to deeper levels.

Reiki

This millennia-old technique was revived in 1920 by a Japanese monk. Like many of those described so far, it focuses on the body on an energetic level. In reiki, the practitioner is said to channel energy using his or her hands and helps the body to regain its balance.

Psychotherapy

In some cases, this is the ideal time to begin psychological therapy, for several reasons: first because we have more time to connect with ourselves. We can therefore more easily access our emotions and feelings, and survey them. Furthermore, if you believe – as I do – that the appearance of a tumour and other diseases has extremely deep-rooted psychological causes, psychological treatment will help to discover and work on the key problem. Whatever therapy you choose (there are also multiple options here, such as Jungian, Freudian, Lacanian, behavioural, or gestalt therapies) it will always help you to better know yourself and to grow. You will neither waste time nor money. However, do not forget that what we are searching for at this time and through all these tools is our improved wellbeing and to make our tumour experience easier. If any of the decisions we make or alternative therapies we undergo in parallel leads us into a black hole, we should leave it aside for the time being.

Chapter Six

THE IMPORTANCE OF NUTRITION

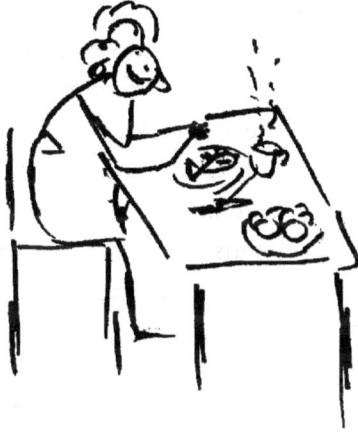

Just as I have devoted an entire chapter to conventional therapies and another to complementary or alternative therapies, I consider that nutrition, given its importance and impact on our health, also merits a chapter of its own.

There are innumerable books that address the subject of food as a source of toxins or with healing properties. And countless schools and options have sprung up around this question.

Each time I visited Master Jin, he gave me some guidelines on what to eat and what to avoid. And I followed them, of course. The truth is that between his and my nutritionist's recommendations the variety of my menus was rather limited. But I didn't mind too much. I knew it was a temporary measure.

Firstly, it's very important to have in mind our dietary considerations before and during treatment and, furthermore, once we understand the impact nutrition has on the body and its ability to both cure and promote the development of illness, we should all consider nutrition as one of our lifestyle changes when our treatment is finalized.

From the moment you begin treatment for the tumour, regardless of the kind you choose, a number of mechanisms are triggered that bring about changes in the body. I refer not only to treatments like chemotherapy or radiotherapy, but also to other natural therapies that address this situation. If we start with a treatment that seeks to eliminate toxins from the body this also promotes changes.

Conventional treatments, whether chemotherapy, radiotherapy, and even surgery, are extremely aggressive. Clearly their goal is to destroy the tumour, but these treatments have a strong impact on the body in the form of collateral damage, which we need to minimize. Our cells and vital organs suffer wear and tear; they weaken as a result of the characteristics of the drugs themselves that destroy healthy cells, and because of the immense effort placed on the body's organs to filter out so many drugs and surmount the treatment. By following a good diet we can make it easier for our body to access the nutrients it needs, instead of giving it more work. Thus, our body will expend less energy, suffer less wear, and we will feel better during the treatment. In short, our recovery will be faster and easier, as it will be shorter.

The extra strain put on the liver or kidneys, for example, due to chemotherapy, not only implies that these organs double their work rate to metabolize new substances, but do so under more extreme conditions, surrounded by toxic elements. Therefore, the healthier and 'cleaner' these organs are from the beginning, the better able they will be to stand up to the challenge.

A cyclist climbing a mountain pass, or a tennis player competing in a long and important final, need at some point in the race or match enough energy to maintain their high level of endurance. And neither of them would think of eating a heavy meal however weak they may feel. We can draw a similar parallel for your body, which is likewise being pushed to the limit, though we don't notice because our liver and kidneys don't hurt, don't warn us. So it's best to make it easy for them. During the treatment period we should simplify our food intake, avoiding fats and sauces, heavy dishes, precooked foods, and so on. Of course, there is no need to feel like we are making a sacrifice. Food is a pleasure that we need not renounce.

Some patients lose a good deal of weight during treatment, especially during chemotherapy.

This is not necessarily due to a lack of food, but because the body needs more energy to metabolize the many chemicals it is receiving. Other people, however, become bloated precisely because their body, sensing a different and extreme situation, reacts by accumulating energy. It's storing up in case the situation persists. Generally our body retains more liquids, and behaves differently to that which we are accustomed.

I decided to eliminate once and for all some foods from my diet. I had wanted to take the plunge for some time and never seemed to find the right moment. I lacked the determination to stand by my decision. My tumour led me to seek more information, to better understand the impact of food on our bodies and our planet, and I became definitely convinced of what I wanted to do, and how and why. Plus, before long I began to feel the benefits of my new diet.

There are no big secrets to a healthy diet. Today everyone talks about healthy eating, though we often still find it difficult to understand the reasons behind it.

I banished from my life refined flour, wheat, dairy products and meat. I hardly ever eat sweet things, and when I do, they are home-made. Obviously, I try not to go to extremes. I followed a very strict diet during the treatment, but over time I've relaxed my regimen a little and if I travel, for example, I adapt to the place I'm in, trying not to be obsessive.

Moreover, I have internalized my new diet to such an extent that it takes no effort to follow it. On the contrary, I greatly enjoy it. The eggs, fruit and vegetables I buy are normally organic, the fish, usually small in size (which accumulates fewer heavy metals, mainly mercury); the flour, also organic, is wholegrain and made of spelt. Instead of crisps, I enjoy dried fruit snacks, organic walnuts or almonds, either raw or toasted. Sugar (it seems impossible, but it's true) is almost absent from my daily diet, and when I do include it, I take unrefined brown sugar, also organic, or honey. We make our own bread, and even yogurt, occasionally, with sheep's milk.

So, why all these changes? What impact does food have on the body if I can't even feel the difference between digesting a sugar-coated pastry dipped in coffee and a slice of spelt bread with extra virgin olive oil and green tea? To respond to these questions, I have taken as a starting point the physiological causes that provoke the emergence and development of a tumour, in order to analyze, from there, how we can change said environment through nutrition.

Addressing the physiological causes related to tumour development through nutrition

All disciplines that study the causes behind the emergence of tumours – whether conventional or alternative therapies, highly medicalized or natural – agree that there are several internal factors that favour the development and reproduction of a tumour cell.

Under normal situations, when our body is in balance, it is able to neutralize and eliminate the defective cells it generates. But when this balance is disturbed, tumour cells can overpower the healthy ones because the environment in which they live is suitable for them to reproduce, whereas it's not apt to host healthy cells.

What we eat plays a fundamental role in this process. It's one of the key means we have at our disposal to modify the habitat of our cells. If we create a balanced environment that facilitates the proper functioning of our body, our cells, and our defences, we can fight the disease at its root. Below, we survey the most important factors that come into play when imbalances take place in the body, in order to understand how we can have some leverage on them.

The immune system

Our immune system is able to halt the growth of cancer cells in the body and eliminate them. It does this hundreds of times in a person's lifetime, although the body does not perceive it. Sometimes our healthy cells are not strong enough to eliminate tumour cells in their initial stages, and that is when the tumour develops and grows.

The immune system can be affected by external and internal agents. Stress, distress and anxiety play a part in lowering our defences. Good nutrition helps our system to recover. While some companies label certain foods as antistress (dark chocolate, for example, which can help reduce and control anxiety levels), we will especially focus on foods that have an impact on the consequences produced on our body by stress, and which keep our immune system healthy.

One of the strongest adversaries against which our defences have to fight are inflammatory processes. Several studies show that tumour progression is closely linked to these processes. Tumour growth functions much like an inflammatory process. Cancer uses this natural inflammation to spread throughout the rest of the body.

Many of the inflammatory processes that occur in our bodies often are preceded and characterized by high doses of stress that undermine our defences. If the immune system is not in top form, it's unable to neutralize and combat cancer cells in the body, and thus these cells begin to take hold. Both factors, the lowering of our defences and the development of internal inflammation, are therefore closely linked.

Food rich in vitamin C (found in many fresh foods, such as broccoli, peppers, citrus fruits, kiwis, etc.) is the immune system's best friend, as it helps to strengthen it. If we add proper oxygenation of the cells to a good dose of vitamins, our defences will be up to the task.

A diet rich in anti-inflammatory compounds that reduces or eliminates the consumption of highly inflammatory products will help us to combat the formation and reproduction of cancer cells in our body. Thus we can help take some of the strain off our immune system and keep it healthy, and it will no longer have to take on and neutralize so many malignant cells, since we will prevent them from forming in the first place. This is why it is so important to incorporate into our diet green tea, extra virgin olive oil, vegetables in general, and foods with high omega-3 levels. All of these have significant anti-inflammatory properties.

Moreover, it is best to avoid eating foods that promote inflammation, such as red meat, sugar and products with saturated fat. In the section dedicated to specific questions you will find this explained in more detail.

Blood pH

Blood pH is another factor to take into account. When your pH is balanced this also stimulates and bolsters the immune system. But more importantly, the fluctuation of pH itself is instrumental in determining whether tumour cells are comfortable or not in the environment they inhabit and, therefore, whether they are strong enough to spread or if they can be blocked.

pH is a measure of alkalinity or acidity. The pH scale ranges from 0 (very acidic) to 14 (very alkaline), and 7 is neutral pH. Our blood is slightly alkaline. Normal reference values range from 7.35 to 7.45.

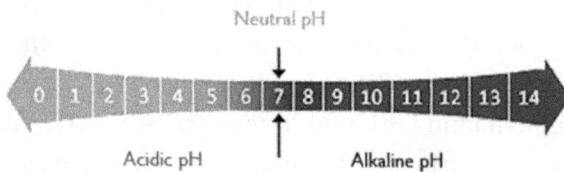

Neutral pH

0 | 1 | 2 | 3 | 4 | 5 | 6 | 7 | 8 | 9 | 10 | 11 | 12 | 13 | 14

Acidic pH   Alkaline pH

Cancer cells proliferate in an acidic environment, which is precisely what harms healthy cells. On the contrary, an alkaline environment promotes the proliferation of healthy cells and inhibits the growth and development of cancer cells.

Food is the natural tool we have at our disposal to keep our pH balanced. Some foods have a high acid content, such as meats, eggs, refined sugars and flours; and others are highly alkaline, as are most vegetables (especially broccoli, garlic, etc.), fruit or green tea. The pH of vegetarians is generally more alkaline than that of the average population because their diet comprises many acidic foods. So proper nutrition also allows you to modify your pH, making it more alkaline and thus combating many diseases naturally.

Annex 2 shows a table that ranks foods according to their impact on our pH.

Lack of oxygen

A highly acidic environment is also poorly oxygenated. Oxygen facilitates the removal of acids from the blood, and thus helps to create a more alkaline environment. This is one good reason to exercise, stay active and breathe deeply. Renewing our body's oxygen makes it more complicated for cancer cells to thrive.

Moreover, properly oxygenated blood strengthens other organ systems, including the immune system. Blood transports nutrients, defences and water. Properly oxygenated blood is healthy and can perform its function normally. Hence, our blood will transport to every corner of our body whatever it needs at that time. If we take care of our blood, it will take care of the rest of our body.

Toxicity

When the body does not function properly, either because it is poorly oxygenated or because its pH is more acidic than it should be, the blood cannot perform its work properly and collect all the waste we produce. Consequently, toxins accumulate in our organs and cells. Among these are the so-called free radicals, molecules that are the result of cellular oxidation and that are produced in the body as a result of stress, smoking, pollution, or poor dietary habits. In excess, free radicals can block natural regeneration and cause cell degeneration.

To combat the accumulation of free radicals in the body we can consume foods that contain a high quantity of antioxidants. There are different types of antioxidants with different characteristics. As it is not my intention to examine this subject in depth, but rather to capture the essence regarding body function, I think it is enough to know of their existence and know where to find them to include them in our diet. Examples of foods rich in antioxidants are nuts, artichokes, broccoli, strawberries, figs, and so forth.

The glycemic index

Lastly, there is another hugely important point to bear in mind if we are to keep our body in balance: cancer cells sustain themselves on the sugar we provide them. A standard blood test will show you how much glucose you have in your blood, and certain kinds of food can lower your glucose levels.

Sugar is found in many foods, not just sweets. Refined flours and pasta, for example, contain abundant sugar; they are composed of carbohydrates that our body processes as glucose.

The *glycemic index* (GI) indicates the speed by which carbohydrates are transformed into glucose. The higher the GI of the food we eat, the greater our blood sugar level.

Food can be classified according to its glycemic index, by taking glucose as a reference, which is given a default value of 100. From there, there are foods with a *low* (under 55), *medium* (55-70) and *high* (more than 70) glycemic index. In order to maintain stable glucose levels, regardless of the type of food we consume, the body (the pancreas, specifically) produces insulin. When you eat foods with a high GI, your body has to counteract high blood sugar levels which produce a steep rise in insulin, called an 'insulin spike'. This creates a vicious circle. We have all experienced the feeling of weakness or dizziness caused by the so-called 'sugar crash'. This sensation is brought on by a lowering of blood insulin levels after the peak. Our body is asking us to maintain the level of the insulin peak, so we introduce more sugar into the system. By ingesting low GI foods, we will maintain a steady level and thereby avoid the need to take sugar because of a slump. This is the best way to prevent our body from resorting to drastic measures.

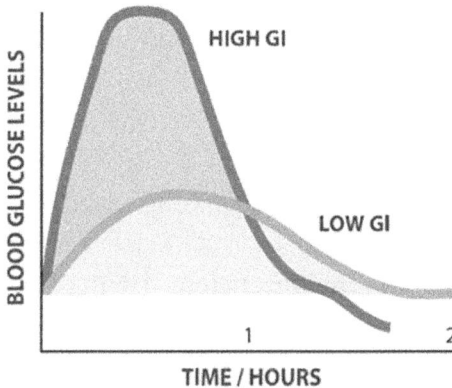

Insulin production is accompanied by the production of a type of protein called IGF (insulin-like growth factor). It is widely documented that IGFs stimulate the tumour cell growth. Therefore, by consuming foods with a high glycemic index, we are creating the ideal breeding ground for the proliferation of tumours. The more insulin produced, the more IGFs present in our body. And the more IGFs there are in the blood, the more food the tumour cells will have to grow and move freely throughout the body.

There is a belief that our brain needs sugar to function. Indeed we do need glucose but as part of a balanced diet. By following the guidelines set out in this book we will obtain the right amount of glucose we need. We mustn't give our body extra sugar. Annex 3 contains a list of foods classified according to their glycemic index.

Roughly speaking, glucose is present primarily and fundamentally in sweets, white flour, starches, pasta, dairy products as well (although the tables indicate otherwise, they behave as if their IG was high) and even fruit, which has large amounts of sugar in the form of fructose.

* * *

Knowing all this, isn't it surprising that hospitals do not give patients dietary guidelines in line with what we have just discussed? We need not feel guilty each time we eat something that's not included in the diet we choose to follow, if we have opted to follow one. But, as always, it is important to be aware of what we do, the reasons and consequences.

By my fourth or fifth cycle of chemotherapy, the nurses, the doctor and I myself had all realized that I had lost a fair bit of weight. I could ill afford to lose any more kilos before starting the next cycle, and between my occasional lack of appetite, the additional energy requirements that my body needed to cope with such an aggressive treatment, and the strict diet I was following, it was logical that I had lost some weight. The nurses, in response to my observations, suggested I might try to eat cannelloni with béchamel sauce, meat and cheese. They said this in all sincerity, with all their love, and this helped me understand how important it is to reach all sectors somehow related to overcoming tumour processes, with sound information about nutrition, so that all of us – patients and health professionals alike – take the same stance.

But returning to the issue of nutrition, if we delve a bit further we shall see that some foods are 'at odds' with one another. Chickpeas, for example, are ideal when taking into account their glycemic index, but they are not suitable in terms of their acidity. Eggs are rich in protein but are also highly acidic. Cold meats and sausages look ideal according to their GI, but we all know that saturated fats are not beneficial since they are also inflammatory and contain cholesterol. Fruit contains many vitamins and antioxidants but, on the other hand, its GI is high. Oily fish provides plenty of omega-3, which is essential, but it's acidic. So what to do? Well, the answer is not to abuse of any particular food. However, instead of adopting the popular concept of 'Eat a bit of everything for a balanced diet', I think we have given ample reasons to show that a good diet does entail leaving out certain things.

Answers to specific questions

Why is it best to avoid sugar?

We know that tumours feed on sugar. Furthermore, sugar spikes cause insulin peaks that go hand in hand with the production of a specific growth hormone that promotes the development of cancer tumours. Since it's very difficult to give up sweets, allow me to propose some alternatives that we can incorporate into our daily diet. Our goal is to reduce the consumption of sugar to a minimum, especially white sugar.

Alternatives

Stevia

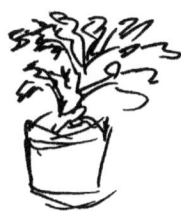

The green leaves of this South American plant are much sweeter than sugar. The GI of stevia is zero, and it's completely natural. Stevia is available as tablets or liquid extract, both of which can be bought from herbalists. The plant itself, either fresh or dried, is on the market as well. Stevia can be grown at home and used just like any other herb. It can substitute sugar in cooking and be used as a sweetener in all kinds of drinks and cakes.

Agave syrup

Also known as agave nectar, it is a golden-coloured molasses that is more liquid than honey. It is extracted from agave, the same cactus which is used to make tequila. This syrup is characterized by its low GI and its high sweetening properties. Agave syrup is used like honey.

Panela

This is the purest sugar, as it is obtained from the juice of sugar cane, which is boiled at high temperatures to produce the liquid. The resulting crystals are panela, which retains all its properties intact. It is the first step to producing brown sugar (which is often just white sugar with molasses extract added to give it a dark appearance). Panela is widely consumed in South America, where it goes under different names: *rapadura, raspadura, chancaca* or *piloncillo*. Being unrefined, panela contains more nutrients than regular sugar does.

Honey

There are many different types of honey (polyfloral, lavender, chestnut, thyme, and so forth). You should buy the high quality, eco-friendly type. Supermarket honey is often manipulated and less pure. Refined sugar is often added, giving the honey a higher IG, which robs it of many of its therapeutic and medicinal properties.

Why reduce our meat consumption?

It's common knowledge that people who don't eat meat have a lower risk of developing cancer and a number of other diseases. Apart from all the studies that corroborate this, it's logical for the following reasons:

> ➤ Meat is acidic. Therefore it contributes to creating an acidic pH in our body.

- Meat is rich in fats, many of which have inflammatory characteristics, so it is best to avoid meat.
- For animals to survive and grow in captivity (often at an accelerated rate), they are injected with antibiotics, tranquilizers, hormones and all kinds of chemicals that eventually enter our body when we consume meat.
- If in addition these meats are smoked or cured, they contain salt, nitrates and nitrites, substances that increase the risk of tumours.
- Moreover, animals bred for consumption are usually raised in a hostile environment. There's little doubt that if we saw how a mass-production chicken farm is run we would give up eating poultry. These animals suffer and this affects the quality of their meat.
- Furthermore, if we want to be environmentally responsible, it is important to have in mind that meat production is largely to blame for the greenhouse effect and all its consequences. If we reduced or eliminated meat from our diet, the level of CO_2 in the atmosphere would drop, a necessary step to reverse global warming. We would all benefit. According to the Food and Agriculture Organization of the United Nations (FAO), producing 1 kg of meat requires 7 kg of grain and 15,000 litres of water (10 times more than is needed to produce 1 kg of grain). Can you imagine how far this water and this grain could go in the fight against hunger?

Alternatives

Meat is an important source of protein. In order to replace it, it's important to choose food that also provides protein. We can always substitute a fillet steak for fish or an omelette. But there are other well-known options for vegetarians, which you may not be as familiar with if you're used to traditional cuisine.

Legumes or pulses

Combined with grains, they provide us with very high-quality protein. Lentils with rice, chickpeas served with a little bread, or barley, oats, millet, beans, etc. These are all very good choices and while they have always been considered as a starter, their high nutritional value means they can be turned into a main course or a single-course meal.

Seaweed

This is an important source of complete vegetable protein. Legumes and pulses need grains to form a complete or high quality protein (equivalent to meat), but seaweed already contains the protein without any need to combine it with other foods. Its use is not yet so widespread, but it's slowly making inroads in a wide range of recipes. It can be added to rice dishes, stews, or beans, and can be consumed on its own and in salads, with a simple dressing.

Seitan

It's made with wheat gluten, which is found in the germ of the seed. Seitan is rich in protein and is cooked in the same way as meat. But beware, it's not apt for celiacs or people who are sensitive to gluten.

Tempeh

This is a paste with the texture of hard custard, made from fermented soya beans. It's rich in protein. Writers such as Andreas Moritz[12] claim that only untreated and properly fermented soya (i.e., at least two years), like tempeh or miso, is fit for human consumption, because this process allows for its digestion. Moreover, soya triggers hormonal processes in our body, so it is not recommended for women who have had a hormone-dependent breast tumour.

---

12. MORITZ, Andreas. *Timeless Secrets of Health & Rejuvenation*. Ener-Chi.com

Tofu

This is not a recommended alternative. Tofu is a hard paste made from soya. It's popular among vegetarians for its high protein content but not all experts are in favour of its consumption. Tofu soya is not previously fermented, so our body cannot digest it. It's important to remember the correlation between soya and hormone production. Women who have developed a breast tumour should also avoid eating it.

Why should we eliminate common wheat from our diet?

Wheat is a modern grain which undergoes various processes to make it more profitable, more productive and more resilient. Many of its properties are lost during this process. Today, wheat has one of the highest glycemic indices (GI) of all foods. Moreover, wheat is largely composed of gluten, ideal for making fluffier doughs but in some cases difficult to digest.

Alternatives

There are many grains that can substitute wheat:

Spelt

An ancient wheat grain which preserves the nutrients that today's wheat has lost, its GI ranks much lower. Furthermore, it does not withstand pesticides very well and is therefore usually organic. It is a good alternative to the wheat flour we normally use. Spelt is also ideal for making dough and bread. It's increasingly easier to find bread made with spelt flour in shops and bakeries.

Kamut

This is the oldest known variety of wheat. Cream coloured, it has a sweet taste and its flour is very fine. The skin of the grain is very thin, which allows it to be cooked like rice. Kamut bread is soft and fluffy, with a sweet touch.

Quinoa

Nutritionally speaking, its properties place it between a grain and a legume. It has high quality protein and is easy to digest. For those who like couscous, quinoa is a good substitute for semolina. It can be eaten cold in salads, and hot with vegetables.

Oats, barley, rye

These grains are rich in nutrients and minerals and offer many possibilities in cooking. Oatmeal is widely used in breakfast cereals. Barley is a good substitute for rice, and rye can be used to make bread that has a somewhat bitter taste.

Why should we not consume white flour and other refined products?

White flour is obtained by separating the grain from its husk and germ, which is the embryo of the seed. The grain is ground, and the husk and the germ – which contain most of the fibre, vitamins and minerals – are discarded or sold separately. These flours are often treated to prevent weevils from forming, or to bleach them. Therefore, they are not pure flours. At present, we do not know what they contain. Moreover, white flours are basically carbohydrates with few nutrients and a very high GI. Hence their outright rejection by all nutritionists, as they have a similar effect on the body to that of sugar.

Why do we find these flours everywhere if their nutritional value is so low? For several reasons, one of them is that they are excellent for cooking. They contain lots of gluten and this makes breads, cakes, and other pastries much fluffier and softer. Another reason is clearly economic: the flours we buy are often made of genetically modified wheat, which is more resistant to pests, and obtains higher yields. The leading international grain producers choose to produce greater quantities for less money at the expense of the product's quality, to exploit the lands beyond the limits of their possibilities, and to manipulate nature itself, creating new grains through genetic manipulation whose impact on our system is still unknown. The sole purpose behind these behaviours is for a chosen few to get rich at the expense of everyone else.

There are many other refined products, such as sugar, which undergo development and transformation processes similar to those described above before they reach us. These products gradually lose their nutrients, have chemicals added to them to make them more aesthetically appealing (the case of some types of brown sugar, which is nothing less than dyed refined sugar) and end up becoming pure glucose, with no other nutritional content than simple energy.

Alternatives to white flour

Any flour that is not refined is a good alternative. Organic flour, by definition, has not been treated or manipulated. Refined flours, however, often contain added products to better preserve them. Spelt flour is the most similar to wheat flour. There is also kamut flour, or rye, which behave similarly to wheat because they all contain gluten.

Another alternative is flour made from rice, corn, quinoa or chickpeas, which you can experiment with in the kitchen. In all cases, it is important to note that pesticides accumulate in the husk of the grain, so if you opt for whole grain flour it should be organic.

Alternatives to refined sugar

This section on sugar above discusses the options available to us.

Which vegetables, fruits, legumes and pulses are the most recommendable?

Some vegetables are considered to have anticancer properties. *Broccoli, onion, garlic and cauliflower* have in common an antioxidant and anti-inflammatory effect, and they regulate pH. It is important to include them in our diet, without fear of consuming too much.

Other foods, such as legumes and pulses, have their pros and cons. We discussed the glycemic index of chickpeas, for example, which are high in protein and have a low GI, yet they are acidic. *Red lentils* are easily digested and have less calories than *chickpeas*. In any case, while these pulses are more acidic than other foods in the tables, they will always be more desirable than meat.

Soya, is also very high in protein, has a low GI and is not acidic, but it is not indicated for people with hormone-dependent breast tumours, since soya components may stimulate the development of these tumour cells. We also mentioned that recent studies advise against soya consumption if it has not undergone a previous fermentation process that makes it digestible.

Seaweed is particularly nutritious. Besides the complete protein it provides, this food contains other essential nutrients, such as calcium, iron, amino acids, trace elements, fibre, etc. It also has antioxidant properties.

Fruits are rich in countless vitamins and fibre, but some, such as pineapple, are considered acidic, and others, such as watermelon, have a high GI. Beyond specific examples we should remember that eating fruit provides high doses of fructose, which is converted to glucose. Therefore, we should eat fruit in moderation. Two or three pieces a day is enough. Fruits containing vitamin C have anti-inflammatory properties. Others, such *as apples*, are regulatory and digestive. They contain lots of fibre, not too much sugar, and can have a healing function both in cases of constipation and diarrhea. *Bananas*, meanwhile, contain a lot of potassium, an important mineral that we sometimes lack.

What about eggs?

Proponents claim that eggs have the highest quality of protein not obtained directly from animal meat. And, moreover, they have a IG of zero.

But, one man's meat is another's poison: egg yolks are acidic, and egg whites are alkaline. And don't forget that eggs contain fat and cholesterol.

On the whole, eggs are an excellent source of nutrition. Until recently consumption was restricted to two or three times a week, because of their high cholesterol content. Today it seems that this amount is flexible because although eggs have cholesterol, if they are of good quality and cooked in a healthy manner, their cholesterol level is not as high as those of any other precooked food that could be used as a substitute.

In terms of quality, this is one of the most variable foods depending on their origin and the treatment of the hens. Eggs from caged hens, fed with feed and refined flour, vary significantly from eggs from free-range hens, which are reared on grain and vegetables. Therefore, it is strongly recommended that you consume organic or free-range eggs, whenever possible.

What about nuts and seeds?

Nuts are similar to fruits. They will be more or less desirable depending on the point of view you take. They are always a good alternative protein, and a good supplement to a diet in which you have restricted your consumption of biscuits, jams, etc.). *Walnuts* are somewhat acidic although the most nutritious of all nuts, and they contain many antioxidants. *Almonds*, meanwhile, are very alkaline and help to regulate our body. The same goes for *cashews, Brazil nuts, tigernuts, hazelnuts* – all of which are very healthy and complete food sources.

Whenever you can, always opt for raw or roasted nuts, without salt or oil. Nuts are often sold fried, with which they lose many of their properties.

Seeds provide an additional food source that we can gradually introduce into our diet. They are rich in fibre, minerals and healthy fats. P*umpkin seeds* and *linseeds*, also called *flax seeds*, for example, contain omega-3; *sesame seeds* are abundant in calcium, protein and vitamin B, so important for the functioning of the nervous system. They can be found in a paste form (called tahini) that can be substituted for butter in our breakfasts. *Sunflower seeds* help to lower cholesterol, and *poppy seeds* contain iron and vitamin A, which has an antioxidant effect.

We can eat them alone, add them to salads, to pie crusts and bread dough, and use them for coating (sesame seeds are ideal) instead of bread crumbs.

Why are so many people against dairy products?

Humans are the only animals that consume milk into adulthood. The rest of mammals consume it only in their first stage of life. Milk is a primary food source, to the point that new-born babies do not need anything else. As we grow, our body evolves, and is able to process more and more foods, but at the same time it loses its natural ability to process others, namely milk. One component of milk is a protein called casein that our body cannot metabolize. Cow's milk contains a higher amount of casein than breast milk. As we grow our body goes through other stages of development and loses its ability to digest breast milk, so what effect does cow's milk have on our stomach?

Most adults don't notice any apparent rejection. We have become accustomed since childhood to consuming so much milk that our body has had to adapt to it, which does not mean that it's easy to digest. In fact, if we study the reactions within our body, we see that milk causes havoc.

One of the most direct and obvious consequences of milk consumption is excessive mucous production. And that doesn't just mean nasal mucus, but also all internal mucus, which in excess hinders digestion by forming a type of paste in the stomach, clogging the intestinal follicles that absorb nutrients, blocking the lungs and creating respiratory problems. What's more, mucus facilitates inflammatory processes in the body.

There are many ways to obtain calcium from foods: nuts are an excellent source of calcium, as are vegetables like spinach, broccoli, cabbage, and so on. There is no need to resort to dairy products for calcium which, furthermore, is also more difficult to assimilate than the calcium we obtain from vegetable produce.

It is interesting to note that many studies show that breast tumour rate is much higher in cultures where dairy products are consumed. Milk promotes the development of estrogen in women. In addition, it provides the body with the same growth hormone that occurs when we experience blood sugar spikes and that, as mentioned above, stimulates tumour cell growth. Add to this the antibiotics that are used to treat animals, and that we ingest through milk, and it's clear that finding alternatives to cow's milk is well worth the effort.

The effect of milk on our body extends to other dairy products, such as cheese, yogurt, cream, etc. If you find it hard to eliminate cow's milk from your diet, you can start by substituting it for milk from smaller animals, like sheep or goats, which is similar to human milk. Sheep's milk curd, for instance, has less of an impact on the body than do yoghurts, and you may also find sheep and goat cheese, which are easier to digest than cheese made from cow's milk.

Alternatives

Luckily, there is a wide range of vegetable milk options to replace animal milks. They can be used in the same manner, both for direct consumption or for cooking. It is advisable to look for options that do not contain any added sugar. There are also cooking creams made

153

from vegetable products that provide a perfect substitute for double or single cream.

Oat milk

It's highly digestible and very complete and provides very good quality protein. Some types contain calcium. It is very mild and a touch sweet. An excellent choice for desserts and cakes and to have at breakfast time.

Spelt Milk

It has gluten, so it may cause intolerance in some people. It also contains protein and it is less sweet than oat milk, making it more suitable for sauces like béchamel and savoury dishes.

Rice milk

Very sweet and mild flavour. In some cases, it may cause constipation.

Quinoa, almond, hazelnut, millet, kamut milk

They can be found in health food shops or stores carrying organic products. All of them are a good choice.

Soya milk

Within the range of vegetable drinks, this is the worst alternative to animal milk. The impact of soya on the body was mentioned when we discussed meat and proteins. It is not recommended for women with hormonal-dependent breast tumours. What's more, transgenic soya beans are used in the production of this drink.

Fats, oil, omega-3 and omega-6 and cholesterol

There is so much talk nowadays about both fats and edible oils that it has become difficult to tell them apart. We read about saturated, unsaturated and hydrogenated fats, about good fats, bad fats, cholesterol, and so on. In the end we get lost.

We can distinguish three basic types of fats.

> **Saturated fats** are natural fats that are solid at room temperature, such as lard, tallow, bacon fat or butter. They tend to raise cholesterol levels, so be careful with them.

> **Unsaturated fats** are oils that are liquid at room temperature. They are essential for the proper functioning of our body. Their absence raises cholesterol levels; therefore consuming these fats help to regulate cholesterol. They are subdivided into:

> * **Monounsaturated** *fats:* found in olive oil, avocado, and some nuts. They lower bad cholesterol and raise good cholesterol.
> * **Polyunsaturated** *fats:* the famous 'omega' fatty acids or substances. The best known are omega-3 and omega-6. There is also omega-9, but less is said about it. They are characterized by their ability to lower bad cholesterol and promote good cholesterol production. It is important to maintain a good balance between the amount of omega-6 and omega-3 in our bodies: four to one. That is, for every four grams of omega-6 we eat, we should consume 1 gram of omega-3. In Western societies the ratio may reach 20 or 30 to one. This imbalance may be responsible for some diseases. Moreover, omega-3 has anti-inflammatory properties, hence its importance for people who have developed a tumour. However, omega-6 is inflammatory and is thus best avoided.

> **Trans fats** or **hydrogenated fats**: liquid fats that have been industrially treated by injecting hydrogen to convert them into solid fats. Manufacturers do this to prevent rapid deterioration

of the product (to stop fried food from going rancid or pastries from hardening). They are extremely harmful, increase bad cholesterol and decrease the good cholesterol.

Regarding *cholesterol*, it is a substance produced by our body, and it is also obtained from the foods we eat. In some cases the body has a deficiency, a productive imbalance, but generally, in people with high cholesterol this imbalance is due to unbalanced nutrition. A balanced intake of unsaturated fats helps to regulate cholesterol.

Fish

There is a wide range of fish, and therefore it can be difficult to make general statements about this food source. It's true that fish is high in protein and easier to digest than meat, and the fat it contains is beneficial to humans. Pay particular attention to the benefits of oily fish and shellfish, as they contain high doses of omega-3, a fatty acid with anti-inflammatory effects.

However, shellfish is generally a highly acidic food, so you should not abuse it so as not to alter blood pH.

Bearing in mind the food chain and the size of the fish we eat, it is always better to opt for small fish (sardines, mackerel, horse mackerel, etc..) rather than big ones (tuna, salmon, swordfish, etc..). Fish accumulate mercury in their bodies and other heavy materials found naturally in the ecosystem and the animals on which they feed. Consequently, most predatory fish such as tuna or swordfish are more toxic than smaller ones.

What about alcohol?

Everyone is more or less familiar with the effect of alcohol on our body, and its high toxicity, especially in the long term. We know it causes cardiovascular disease, which damages the brain and affects many of our vital organs. But these consequences are the result of excessive consumption; even the World Health Organization (WHO) recommends drinking a glass of red wine a day to keep your heart in shape.

However, during chemotherapy treatment it is best to completely eliminate alcohol consumption. Like many other substances, alcohol places huge demands on the body, especially the liver, in order to be metabolized. And we've seen that the liver is already under great strain during treatment. It will accumulate work, so to speak; it is therefore much better to facilitate its functioning as much as possible.

Once we have recovered from treatment, what should our ideal relationship be with alcohol? Is it better to have that glass of wine recommended by the WHO, or not? The Million Women study conducted by the Oxford University[13] shows that women who consume alcohol in moderation (one drink several times a week) are more likely to develop a tumour. There is also research (Cedars-Sinai Medical Center, Los Angeles[14]) that claims otherwise. Alcohol has inflammatory characteristics, so from my point of view it is better to opt for occasional consumption.

That said, as I always point out, each of us must learn to take responsibility for our diet, and obviously, for our own body.

---

13. Moderate Alcohol Intake and Cancer Incidence in Women. JNCI J Natl Cancer Inst (2009) 101 (5): 296-305 first published online February 24, 2009 doi:10.1093/jnci/djn514.
    http://jnci.oxfordjournals.org/content/101/5/296.full.pdf
14. Red Versus White Wine as a Nutritional Aromatase Inhibitor in Premenopausal Women: A Pilot Study: Chrisandra Shufelt et al. Journal of Women's Health. March 2012, 21(3): 281-284.
    http://online.liebertpub.com/doi/abs/10.1089/jwh.2011.3001

Chapter Seven

SOME REMEDIES TO TACKLE THE SIDE EFFECTS OF TREATMENTS

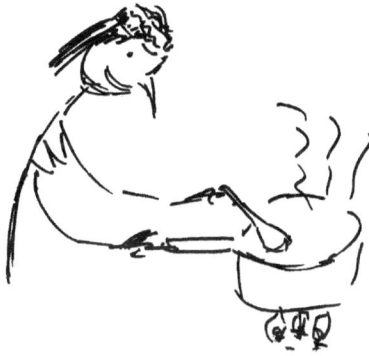

The most important idea that I think we should keep in mind throughout the entire treatment is *all things pass and everything comes to an end.*

Why? Because one of the things I've achieved through chemotherapy is to exercise a little patience. I recognize that as the chemo becomes a distant memory, my characteristic impatience – which has accompanied me since my earliest memories, together with my haste to get to more things done in less time – is once again vying for the position it enjoyed in my 'former life'. But I don't allow it. I now recognize it and will not let this impatience re-establish itself and have free reign. Even as a child I would run to the school bus stop because I spent every last minute in a rush. This has been my way of life. Always do a little more, a little faster and a little better. And in the end, all for what? It's no big deal if something is left undone, or if we do it tomorrow. I suppose I took too seriously the adage "don't leave for tomorrow what you can do today", and I twisted it around to the point that my goal was to do everything today to have nothing pending tomorrow.

Obviously, and thankfully, this will not be the point of departure for all of us. And yet, it's still important to remember that *all things pass, it's just a matter of time.* The body is wise, from the moment we let it start to regain its balance it will surprise us. It always does. Even if we are forced to make decisions that leave a deep physical imprint, such as the removal of a breast, or if we suffer after-effects such as lymphedema – which we will discuss – or sensitivity to sunlight. The body will also know how to recover with time and affection; little by little, it will find a way to adapt to the changes, and the new situation won't be as terrible as that which we initially envisaged.

> *The body is wise: once we let it start to regain its balance it will surprise us.*

Yes, I know. I know very well that when you just get out of the operating theatre, or when your defences are at rock bottom and you cannot even climb two steps, everything seems impossible, and I know my words ring hollow. They are not new. Nurses and doctors also repeat them, though they help little. Hopefully the voices of everyone who has been through this will help to address the moment with optimism and above all, I insist, with patience.

When a friend described to me the chemotherapy she had undergone, before I started mine, she said, "You'll notice how it accumulates: During the first cycle (the first 'fix', shall we say) the first few days are the worst, then they get better, and during the third week you'll feel okay. But, as you have more chemo sessions, you'll find that the period in which you feel bad gets longer, it becomes more difficult to recover and you don't feel as strong when you begin the next cycle."

I appreciate her words and her love. I had them in mind, perhaps too much, because I was slightly conditioned by this advice when

I started the process. And while it's true I experienced tough times during the chemo treatment, I recovered well from all the cycles. It was not a bleak year in which I was homebound. It was a year full of new experiences, of novelties and of hitherto unknown feelings. The chemotherapy allowed me to relax, to stop doing what I thought everyone expected of me, to let go of being there for others as I (not them) thought I should be. I stopped demanding so much of myself, because I needed to focus my energy on more pressing needs, such as staying active, being in a good mood, helping out at home and keep going to the cinema from time to time. And what peace!

Another friend, who was taking her mother to chemotherapy, recounted a conversation she had with a patient who said, "What can I say? I'm overjoyed with this chemo, for once in life I do nothing at home. My husband does everything and I let him take care of me." So you see, there are many ways of addressing these months.

Fundamentally, with chemotherapy treatment it's quite possible you will perceive many changes. Some of these you will have heard about, and others will be new. Each body reacts differently to the treatment. Be patient. Try not to despair. Remember: all things pass.

That said, let's review some tips and remedies that can help us through difficult times.

I have nausea and digestive problems

Nausea is habitually associated with chemotherapy treatments. Although the treatment itself includes cortisone to reduce this sensation, it is not always possible to entirely eliminate it. Here are a few suggestions that can provide some relief:

Marijuana Oil

Obviously, it has its supporters and detractors. My Chinese doctor didn't agree with its use, so after having obtained all the material I needed to make the oil – I had even cooked the first batch – I put it in a drawer and never got to try it. But it was a tremendous help for lot of people I know. They used it as a salad dressing, or on toast, always raw. And it offered relief.

Recipe

You need a handful of marijuana, preferably the plant buds, and half a litre of extra virgin olive oil. Heat the marijuana in a bain-marie for half an hour, stirring so it does not boil (it's important that the temperature of the oil does not rise above 70°C, as the marijuana will lose its properties). Allow it to macerate for 24 hours and strain. The oil is now apt for consumption. One tablespoon a day is enough to feel its effects.

Ginger

This root is widely used by pregnant women during the first months of pregnancy. Its use as a spice is very common in Asian countries. Ginger relieves nausea and vomiting and transmits heat to the body. It can be eaten in many ways. It can be taken as an infusion, by boiling the root, or eaten raw in food, both in salads and in casseroles. It's worth incorporating into your daily diet during chemo, because it replenishes and helps you feel better.

If you don't like its strong and spicy taste, you can take it in capsule and tablet form, preferably organic.

Recipe

To make a cup of *ginger tea* you will need a small root, which you should chop and then boil for 10 minutes. Let stand for a few minutes, then strain, and it's ready for drinking. Ginger tea helps to conduct body heat in cold weather.

Another way of consuming this root is by preparing *ginger water*. Grate the ginger directly into hot water with a dash of lemon. One glass in the morning, in a fasting state, helps to eliminate toxins from our body and it does not take as much preparation time as an infusion.

Other Alternatives

Many people find that *cola beverages* help. Though not the ideal choice, due to their high sugar content, there are times when we cannot rule out any option.

Acupuncture is another way to relieve these symptoms.

If nothing else calms us, we can try *herbal relaxation pills*, like those made with valerian. They help you get through the day in a mellow state of drowsiness. Thus, gradually the nausea will subside and two or three days after the last cycle we will no longer notice it. This was the option that best worked for me. I am very sensitive to nausea, and the pills I was prescribed at the hospital did not work.

The ginger and acupuncture somewhat alleviated the nausea, but they did not stop the symptoms. So the best I could do was to muster all my patience and wait for the days to pass.

Moreover, you should take care of your stomach to aid digestion and restore intestinal flora that is lost. You can use *stomach protectors*, preferably those made with natural products. There is one such product made from aloe vera that is sold in sachets and works very well. If this product is difficult to find, you can use aloe vera juice on its own.

To maintain *intestinal flora* there are also some natural products that help repopulate the digestive ecosystem. These are probiotic products containing bacteria that are lost as a result of chemotherapy, and are essential for proper digestion and to better absorb nutrients.

I don't know what to eat. Nothing appeals to me

Lack of appetite is a direct consequence of nausea. If you don't feel like eating, it's best not to force your body during the first few days; let the critical moment pass, as we discussed in the section above.

When it's time to sit down for a meal, we can choose bland foods without sauces: poached white fish, vegetable broth, apple compote (see recipe), steamed vegetables, etc. Hospitals recommend yogurt. My proposal is to use *cereal-based desserts* of oatmeal or almond (not soya).

Recipe for apple compote

Wash and peel the apples. Cut into small pieces and put in a pot. Add a bit of lemon juice to prevent the fruit from oxidizing and retain their nutrients, a cinnamon stick or powdered cinnamon and, if you wish, grated or chopped ginger. Pour one or two inches of water into the pot and leave to cook on a slow heat for 20 to 30 minutes. Stir the compote now and again, and add water if it has evaporated. As your appetite returns, you can introduce Budwig cream into your diet.

Budwig cream

Dr Johanna Budwig (1908-2003) was a German biochemist who developed a complex and extensive protocol for healing, fundamentally through nutrition. She realized that most diseases had their causes in four factors:

- The accumulation of toxins in our body
- A weak immune system
- An acidic pH
- Oxygen deprivation

From this starting point, Dr Budwig investigated how different foods and their combinations could, in adequate amounts, cause changes in the body to the point of achieving a cure. She developed a diet based on the intake of omega-3 fatty acids, fruits and fresh vegetables, and her famous *Budwig cream*, based on a combination of fatty acids and proteins.

Budwig always stressed the need to prepare the cream for immediate consumption, and to use exactly the ingredients she specified, as it is the fusion of its components that causes changes at the molecular level (it facilitates oxygenation of body tissues and cells and is absorbed quickly).

Budwig Cream Recipe

Today this recipe has been revised and there are several variations, such as using vegetable rennet instead of cottage cheese.

I thought it would be appropriate to include a recipe with variations. But it is important for the ingredients to be organic and high quality, and for the oils to be first cold-pressed.

Ingredients
- 3 teaspoons of yogurt or low-fat cheese (20%). You can use vegetable rennet
- 2 teaspoons of linseed, wheat germ or sunflower oil
- Juice of half a lemon
- 2 teaspoons of dried nuts or seeds, raw and freshly ground (sesame, linseed, pine nuts, pumpkin seeds or sunflower seeds, almonds, hazelnuts, etc.)
- 3 teaspoons of raisins or ½ ripe banana, or 2 dried figs, or 3 prunes
- 2 teaspoons of raw, ground-in-the-moment cereal (oats, millet, rice, barley, spelt, rye or buckwheat)

First emulsify the oil with yogurt or vegetable curd by beating the mixture for 10 minutes. Add the remaining ingredients. Serve Budwig cream with an infusion and seasonal fruit.

Dry skin and mucous membranes

Dryness of the skin and mucous membranes varies from one person to another. It took me a long time to notice how dry my skin had become, maybe because I've always moisturized my body. It was most clearly perceptible in my face. The dryness, combined with my weight loss, deepened my lines and furrows, and new wrinkles appeared. It seemed as if I had suddenly aged five years. But this, like many other things, also disappears. Your face recovers its smoothness and healthy tone. There are some tricks that can help us. I prefer to use very hydrating, natural products that promote cell regeneration. Creams containing chemical products place extra demands on the body, for they penetrate the skin and force the body to work twice as hard to metabolize these products and also to eliminate the toxins. There is much controversy concerning this issue, as opponents of parabens (substances already discussed) believe that the body is unable to metabolize all the chemicals it absorbs and as a result they accumulate in our tissues, causing diseases, specifically breast cancer. When we refer to the use of oils, we refer only to organic and first cold-pressed oils. Only then will we ensure that their properties are not altered.

Oils for the skin

If your tumour is hormone-dependent, avoid rose hip oil. Rose hip contains the hormone estrogen that feeds hormone-dependent tumours. Alternatively, you can use wheat germ oil, which is also highly moisturizing and regenerative thanks to its vitamin E content.

For the body

Mix wheat germ oil and macadamia nut oil in equal parts. The resulting oil is perfect for daily body moisturizing after your shower, on either wet or dry skin.

For the face

If your complexion is very dry, in the morning mix a few drops of wheat germ oil in rose water and apply it gently. Then leave it to dry. Repeat the procedure at night, even using the oil directly, without diluting it with water. Wheat germ oil is sensitive to sunlight, so undiluted it's best used at night. Avoid applying directly to the eyelids, because it makes them heavy.

For scars

Once the surgical wound has closed, we can help it to heal by directly applying wheat germ oil. Pure aloe vera gel may also be included in the treatment, since it is a potent regenerator. You can repeat the application up to four or five times a day.

For the mouth

Sores or ulcers may appear. This happened to me suddenly, upon changing treatment. I had two difficult days when I was unable to eat because of the pain. Moreover, I also had to deal with a fungal infection which developed in my mouth and windpipe. Gargling with water and thyme, made as an infusion, prevents and relieves mouth sores. Another option, which should not be abused because it can damage tooth enamel, is to gargle with water and baking soda after brushing our teeth. Both products help to disinfect. After oral cleaning, aloe vera can be directly applied to the gums. Aloe vera can also be consumed as juice or syrup, which cleanses and soothes the windpipe and will help to fight fungal infections of the mouth. There are also pharmacy products that soothe gum irritation and canker sores. The treatment of fungal infections is usually long and requires the use of fungicides. The natural remedies we've seen do help, but once the fungal infection has taken hold, they are often insufficient so you will need to resort to medications. Standard therapy is to take a syrup after every meal for weeks, even months. So it's best to take preventative measures to avoid having to go to extremes.

For the eyes

If one day you wake up in the morning and find your eyelids are stuck together, or if your eye suddenly becomes itchy for no apparent reason, you probably have dry eyes. It can occur at any time once you've started chemotherapy. So it's best to avoid this situation by hydrating your eyes before they demand it themselves. This advice is particularly aimed at people who have never had eye problems, as they find it harder to understand the language in which our eyes speak, and understand that this is how our eyes tell us they are dry. The simplest solution is to use artificial tears, sold in pharmacies, that can be used as often as needed. At the height of my chemo I was using this product three or four times a day. Even now I need to use it in the morning, I don't know if it's because I'm used to it or because I really have a drier conjunctiva. Artificial tear products are basically composed of water, without chemical agents. Their composition varies. In some cases, those bought in the pharmacy contain preservatives and stabilizers. Some commercialized artificial tears are made with entirely natural and homeopathic products, which are a very good option, although they are more expensive and difficult to find.

For the vaginal area

The vagina can also become affected by dryness. It may often feel itchy and less lubricated. You might even note a loss of flexibility in this area. Fungal infections or small wounds may develop in the vagina. One way to help our bodies during this period is to provide it with the body's natural flora that serves as a defence against infection and external aggressions. Chemotherapy also attacks the genital area, as well as other rapidly dividing cells. There are capsules (or pessaries) that are completely natural, which are inserted vaginally over ten consecutive days. They are a combination of probiotics that regenerate vaginal flora and have no contraindications. It's one of those products that are worth using from time to time, no need to wait until starting treatment or becoming sick to utilize it. An extra supply of these microorganisms will help us to protect ourselves better and maintain balanced flora. They are found in any pharmacist that stocks natural products. There are also some intimate oils and soaps that help to moisturize, protect from yeast infections and soothe itching. These products often contain a mixture of disinfecting essential oils, including tea tree. They also serve as a vaginal lubricant during intercourse. It's worth mentioning the subject of sex, because tumour treatments tend to affect this aspect of our lives for several reasons: the first is that if you're tired, you probably will not feel like having sexual relations as usual. The second reason is that maybe you do, but your body does not respond. And the third is that you may start having negative thoughts, going into a dangerous spiral of believing you are no longer as attractive as before because you have changed slightly. There are probably more reasons, but they do not come to mind. These three are sufficiently important in themselves. And if during the process we find ourselves in one of these situations, I think it's good to remember once again that they are transitory.

True, vaginal dryness may take a while to rebalance. You will not be as fresh the day after the last session of chemo. But, with time, and by applying the remedies I've mentioned, you will notice significant recovery. Moreover, this may be a good time to explore a new approach to sex, more foreplay. Penetration is not essential, it's only one part of sex that can be reached after foreplay and petting.

I'm tired. I don't feel like doing anything

There are two types of fatigue: physical, when the body doesn't respond, and psychological, which can be experienced as self-neglect, loss of interest in things, and the like.

It's alright to listen to your body and not exert it if it asks you for rest. But if you let yourself sink into apathy and feel a lack of desire to do things, when your body does begin to respond it will be more difficult to recover. It's a vicious circle: the less you move, the less you want to move. One should maintain a minimum of movement, take part in activities and even alternative therapies that help us to socialize and keep in good condition.

Simply getting up in the morning and having a shower can sometimes become something of a challenge. It's alright to admit this. And it's okay to do it every day, routinely. It's the way to get going and prepare for the new day, overcoming weakness. Having a short stroll, going out to buy bread, or taking a look at the house plants will help to keep up your spirits. Try to do it every day, because a shower and a walk will ward off that unpleasant feeling of infirmity. Intriguingly, breast tumours don't make you feel bad. It's the treatment that causes these symptoms. It's rather strange and difficult to accept that the treatment makes you feel sick, rather than the illness itself. So if we feel weak it's not that we are ill, but that our body is working over-time to absorb all the substances that are being injected, and trying to recover. We can help it. But how?

On the one hand, by keeping physically and intellectually active. Usually you will have to take time off work. Try to keep doing things that will motivate and amuse you... Write, play an instrument, read, cook, see friends, go to the cinema. It's a good time to do some volunteer work, if you have ever contemplated this. It can be done from home: helping an NGO with their paperwork. It's also a good opportunity to try your hand at painting, if that's what you've always wanted to do, or fill the house with jigsaw puzzles, or make models. If your demands are not too rigorous, it's always good to have something to do to stay busy and feel useful. I think one of the hardest feelings to overcome is to feel a bit of a burden, because you cannot maintain the same rhythm as you did before. The best way to avoid going to pieces is by helping out as much as we can, both in and outside the home.

The treatment is long, and there is no sense in ending up exhausted whenever you get going. When I think of our body dynamics I am reminded of the heating systems of mountain lodges, and how their owners who keep the house shut up for five days and only go up at weekends explain that it's better to leave the heating on very low and keep the house a little warm, rather than try to heat it up all of a sudden when you arrive, because these sharp peaks consume much more energy. The same goes for our body. It's better to keep up constant and daily activity without major fluctuations, without burning oneself out, rather than wait for the third week after treatment, when we feel much stronger, and suddenly start doing all the errands we have pending.

We have seen the importance of food, so we will not discuss this further. What is clear is that the easier we make it for our body, the less energy we will waste trying to digest and process heavy foods. Gentle exercise (walking, swimming, yoga, etc.) will keep our body moving. Blood circulates better, and we will eliminate toxins more easily.

My mind does not work as it did before

To date there has been little discussion about the effects of treatment in terms of the ability to reason, concentrate, analyze things, make decisions and so forth. But they do exist and now they have a name.

In medical terms these effects are known as 'post-chemotherapy cognitive impairment', or 'chemo brain'.

A certain loss of the cognitive function during chemotherapy is considered normal. We are injected with highly aggressive substances that undermine our whole being. I think the best way to cope with this situation is to acknowledge it, not to make a big issue out of not having the same cognitive functions we had prior to treatment.

This lack of concentration may be associated with motor function problems, because our reflexes don't respond as fast as they did before treatment. Thus, for example, it wouldn't be surprising that upon opening a cupboard you bang your head against the door for having miscalculated the distance. It's much easier to catch your finger, bump into furniture, drop things, you get the idea. Sometimes we're only truly aware of the powers we have lost when we've recovered them, because since they disappear little by little, we get used to experiencing these situations as normal. But beware, this is not normal. Some people are not even able to drive, as they are not able to process the many stimuli or their reflexes are not as alert. It's very important to keep this in mind.

As the treatment becomes a distant memory our faculties return to us. We will no longer leave the keys in an impossible-to-remember place in the house, or at least not so often, although some of these symptoms are likely to persist over time. You make a shopping list and leave it at home, take complex and reasoned decisions, then you don't remember what cognitive process led you to make that decision – it's as if, from time to time, the information stored in the brain is inaccessible, as if shrouded in a fog, but somehow you know it's there. It's not a permanent oblivion, because at some point the fog dissipates and you once again remember clearly that reasoning (or the place where you left the keys).

You may experience awkward situations, such as listening attentively to a friend explaining something very personal which after a few days you don't remember. It's easy to say you weren't paying attention, but this isn't true. You were there with your five senses but the information is gone.

Maybe you have trouble remembering the pin code of your credit card (something that never happened before), and when it comes back to you, you're amazed that you could have forgotten it in the first place. You may find it difficult to make associations, or even understand complex film plots. If you know someone elderly who is beginning to suffer lapses of memory, you will surely understand this much better. It may also resemble the situation many pregnant women describe. They experience an apparent loss of attention and difficulties retaining information – memorizing a phone number, for example, can be quite a challenge. Doctors are now beginning to study these side effects, which are not only attributed to chemotherapy. It has been found to be a recurrent side effect in patients who have had breast cancer and Hodgkin's disease, mainly because these patients, who have a higher and longer survival rate, make a full recovery, yet in the mid- and long-term they continue feeling the negative effects of treatment.

If you experience these or similar symptoms, it's useful to do puzzles, crosswords, games of mental skills, and read. You can also include omega-3 fatty acids in your diet. Don't give up, nor take for granted that it will last a lifetime, because it need not. Many people experience a huge improvement in the second year after treatment. We know that the medication is very aggressive, and our body needs time to recompose itself. So it's best to give yourself the time you need, not let it overwhelm you or get you down.

Weird things happen to me. Other side effects

Other less familiar side effects may occur.

Loss of vision

Trying to focus is perceived as a major challenge when you are tired and the small print is not as sharp to you as before. You usually recover your sight after a while. These symptoms may overlap with the onset of presbyopia – commonly known as eyestrain or tired eyes – from the age of forty. It's best not to worry about it and allow a few months to pass after treatment before visiting an optician for an eye test.

Loss of nails

This doesn't happen in all chemotherapies, and nor does it happen to everyone. Furthermore, the intensity varies greatly. Some people lose the entire nail, and others just part of it. Some people's nails turn yellow and opaque, as occurs in the elderly. Make sure your nails are well cut, and if they become fragile, cover them with surgical tape to prevent them catching on the objects you touch. Little else can be done. Avoid manicures to prevent injury and infection, but there's no problem in painting them to lend a touch of colour!

Tingling sensation in the extremities

This symptom may accompany the loss of nails described above, but not always. Sometimes nerve endings are altered due to treatment and your fingers, toes and palms may feel numb and stiff. You should keep them active by doing moderate exercise, walking, opening and closing your hands and even massaging them. The feeling usually disappears, but recovery is slow. In my case, the soles of my feet still feel rather numb and lack flexibility, and my fingers are not as sensitive as they were before, but they have improved a lot since I first noticed these symptoms during treatment. Now it's mostly a shadow of what it was, something I've got used to and therefore give it no importance.

Saliva

It's one of those rare and annoying side effects. It's also poorly documented, and there is no medication to combat it. I know of only one other situation that causes excessive salivation, and that's during pregnancy. It may begin immediately after you have been given the medication, and it doesn't necessarily occur during the first cycle of chemotherapy. It abates after some days, until it's completely brought under control. Chewing gum is one way to control excessive salivation, but there are times that it's so intense the only solution is to carry a handkerchief or go and spit it out in the sink.

Lack of coordination

It's not unusual to find yourself slow, maybe you collide with cupboards and furniture more often. Your reflexes don't respond as they used to, and it's hard to move. But knowing that it's a only consequence of the medication helps you to cope with it naturally.

Emotionality and other feelings

You will very likely feel more sensitive, more vulnerable. Also, sometimes you may get trapped in obsessive thoughts to which you would have previously come up with an immediate solution. Chemotherapy can sometimes deprive you of your resources for dealing with everyday situations: a simple phone call to the cleaners, for example, can be a major effort. We feel far more insecure. It's also possible that people's trivial remarks may bother or hurt you. We feel especially vulnerable, and we may cry more easily, we feel alone, misunderstood or unhappy. These are moments of fragility, often a result of the chemo. But they are side effects, and they also go away. The memory remains, which is fortunate because you start to realize that you are returning to your normal self, and those tasks that formerly seemed impossible are once again trivial transactions.

Chapter Eight

LIFE DURING TREATMENT. SMALL VICTORIES

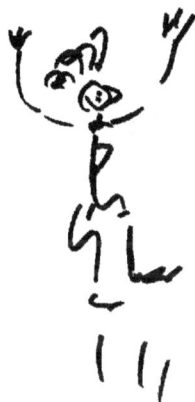

By now you may be wondering, "Why was I not told all this?" Well, often because the people around you don't have access to this information. No matter how much you study in books, life's true teacher continues to be experience itself. Moreover, much of the information I have shared in these pages comes from a wide range of sources and not the purely scientific knowledge which is routinely used in the Western world and taught in schools. We learn biology, natural sciences and mathematics from an early age, yet we are not taught about the close relationship between the body, emotions and mind. We don't learn that our feelings mark us physically. Nor are we taught how energy – so essential for the proper functioning of our body and of our psyche – flows through us. Or how disruptions in this energy flow give rise to health imbalances.

These alternative sources of knowledge to which I refer are not necessarily less valid for being less known. They are different options that, although relegated to the background, are as accessible as conventional medicine. We just need someone to tell us where to start.

Regardless of your progress in negotiating the different stages of the road, one thing is certain: the process will be long. So it's important to be thankful for the small achievements, to celebrate and keep in mind that after each stage there is less to go. If you have a cycle every three weeks, take advantage of the third week to enjoy yourself. Go to that restaurant you've had on your list, meet up with a friend, go to the cinema, have a walk – don't isolate yourself, don't think about the next session of chemo. Try to just enjoy each day without letting despondency prevail. Life will surprise you with small and not-so-small gifts.

Two or three days after my first chemo session, I managed to leave the house wearing my hair montage and neckerchief. I remember it was a sunny day, so I put on a pair of sunglasses. I was wearing jeans and a T-shirt, and I had put on a little makeup because I was starting to look noticeably pallid. I was feeling neither good nor bad, just strange: I felt I had 'undergoing chemo' written all over my face, and that everyone was looking at me and knew it – until I passed some builders who were working at street level. Suddenly... they wolf-whistled at me! It had been years since someone last did that at me in the street. I was so surprised, so thankful; I burst out laughing with joy. I could hardly contain myself. So I phoned a friend there and then to tell her, and we laughed together. It was a real adrenaline rush. I felt beautiful and self-confident. It made me smile to think what one has to go through in order to have someone wolf-whistle their approval at you!

I was aware of my own reaction, so positive. And I thought that if I had reacted differently, which could have happened, I wouldn't have felt so euphoric. I could have been angry, having taken their indulgence as sexist, or I could have ignored it. Instead I decided to enjoy it to the fullest. I mention this to stress once again the importance of maintaining a positive approach towards life in general. This experience helped me to understand how my own attitude could change the way I experienced that occurrence and allow me to squeeze every last drop out of it.

Another wonderful recollection began one Sunday lunchtime. We had arranged to meet some friends. One of them had come from Madrid to spend the weekend in Barcelona. After lunch I was supposed to meet two female friends of mine to do a photo shoot (for work) in order to post some photos on a website.

The lunch was great fun. When it was time to head back, my friends accompanied us home, to have a coffee and relax a bit before starting the shoot at the Health Centre where I was collaborating, next to my house.

I got ready, grabbed my cameras, and was about to leave. Joss insisted on coming with me to carry the equipment. It was really not necessary. I didn't know if he was being overprotective, I found it rather odd, but we went together. I arrived to find the two friends whom I had arranged to meet waiting for me and who then accompanied me to the Centre's conference room, where we were to take the photos. Upon opening the door, I found the floor full of lit candles, and was just able to make out the faces of many friends in the half-light, and suddenly two other friends struck up a tune on their koras,[15] there and then.

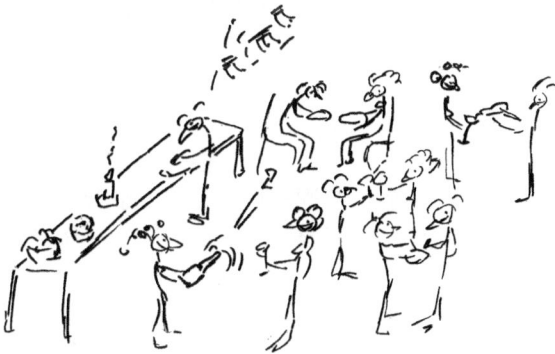

---

15. The kora is a 21-string instrument typical of West Africa. It has a sound similar to the harp, and its music is gentle and soothing.

It was a wonderful party. More than twenty people had come to show me their support and love. I hadn't yet finished the chemo, but they had planned to give me the surprise during my treatment because I was still at a low ebb. On a whiteboard in the room, someone had written in huge letters "We love you, Teresa."

After such a display of affection, one can only give thanks to life, to people, and let oneself get carried away by it all. Other great gifts were to come which I would celebrate in one way or another.

The last chemotherapy session

Though I didn't feel as strong in the last session of chemo as I had in the others, I knew that henceforth I would start to feel better and better.

The end of treatment

This time Joss and I threw the party for all our friends. I think the radiotherapy ended in late July and the party was held in late September.

The day my period came

I suppose this heralded my return to normality, to turning a new page. We went to dinner and celebrated it. This time when I looked at myself in the mirror I smiled, pleased to see that my oily skin had returned. I never thought I'd be so glad to get my blackheads back.

The operation

It marked the end of the toughest part of treatment. Although I would take time to recover, I knew that I no longer had any more hospital appointments ahead of me that made me feel like a used rag.

The last radiotherapy session

The staff was charming in the department where I was treated. They made a real effort to be punctual and to see each patient at their designated time. It went so fast that I barely had time to chat. I never saw a long face or an apathetic look. I suppose it was partly for this reason – since the end of the radiotherapy usually means the end of continuous visits to the hospital – that one feels so grateful and you want to convey it somehow. I made some homemade bread for them as a token of my appreciation, even though I know they're just doing their job, I know it wasn't necessary. It was still warm when I gave it to them and entire ward was steeped in the aroma.

The day I removed my wig

That was a great day. I took pictures to get a good look of myself from all angles before making the big decision and, feeling a trifle insecure, I went out for dinner in a village I'd never been to before, with Joss and some other friends. It was a test but it went so well, I felt so at ease, that I found it impossible to put the Buff with extensions back on my head.

There are many more small victories like I share here. The first steps for me were fundamental. Sometimes when I see people who have been traumatized by their experience with treatment and suffer from their bad luck and ill health, I am saddened that they fail to acknowledge their little triumphs; they see only what is not working as they would wish, that's why they feel so bad.

Chapter Nine

WHEN IT'S OVER: POSSIBLE AFTER-EFFECTS

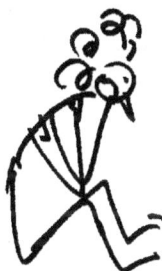

Upon finishing the treatment there is still a lot to do to make a full recovery. Sometimes the after-effects can be long-lasting, permanent even. After everything that the body has been put through over these months, it's logical that it will need at least another two years to regain its balance. During this time, you should maintain some basic care (continue moisturizing your skin, exercise, eat healthy) and observe yourself.

Curiously, throughout the entire treatment process you yearn for things to return to how they were before. You know you'll you need some time to recover and you'll always have a scar on your breast, but you think you can jump back on that same train you got off, and pick up where you left off, doing things as you did before.

In fact, nothing ever goes back to before; it's never like that. Life is constantly changing, especially when we've had intense experiences: we never see reality in the same light after an incredible trip, after changing your job, after meeting your partner or having a child, after graduating from university or moving to another town. Nor do we return to the former life we left behind once the treatment is over, but to a life that has moved on after almost a year. Your whole environment will be one year older. You will obviously have accumulated experiences, memories, a hefty dose of affection and self-confidence – which is enough in itself. You need not go any further and look for more 'meaning' in the experience. Sometimes people will say, "You must have learned a lot", a tribute that may put more pressure on us regarding what is expected of us. It seems that it's not enough to have been through it, we must also have learned from it. Society believes that because you've been at 'death's door' and survived, then you have become a wiser person. But through your eyes, neither did you feel close to death, nor did you accumulate great learning experiences that differed from other stages of your life, nor, of course, do you feel any wiser. All steps give meaning to the path of life and gradually make us wiser. When someone breaks our heart no one asks us if we feel wiser. Why should they do so now? Would there, perchance, be even a hint of 'morbid curiosity' in the idea of risking one's life?

As an executive, I came to address my treatment as just another business project – with a beginning, eight cycles of chemotherapy, surgery, radiotherapy and an end: – that I then filed, and moved on.

However, even though I put a lot of energy into getting my life back on track after treatment, as if the subject really was closed and surmounted, this was not exactly true. My intention was not to hide or deny the tumour I'd had in my breast. I just didn't want my experience to define me to the extent of it conditioning and determining the rest of my life. I didn't want to keep it in mind forever, because I believe that life is a collection of experiences, some more important than others. And having been through this one, I wanted to turn my attention to those that are still to come, many of them wonderful, others probably tough. Curiously, as I gradually put the past behind me, my memory of the process – rather than fade – became more intense.

I finished radiotherapy in late July. In August we were taking a break in the mountains, walking, enjoying the sense of tranquillity and good friends.

During my radiotherapy in July, I asked to have the portacath removed. I had to obtain authorizations from several doctors, as the standard procedure is to leave the portacath in place over the five years of follow-up tests, but in my case we had already reached an agreement with the oncologist that it would be removed. That was my condition for having the portacath implanted in the first place. I wanted to return to my normal life, and one of my normal activities was to go scuba diving, which was incompatible with a catheter. How I needed that! So in September we went on a short diving holiday.

It was a relaxing week. Our only plans for the daytime were eating and diving. It sounded great. I applied several layers of high protection sunscreen and, wearing a hat and long-sleeved T-shirt, I walked around the island until I donned the wetsuit.

Scuba diving does not require great skills and entails little effort. At times one feels hot with the wetsuit on, and the air tank is heavy, but apart from that, it's a peaceful activity.

I was truly leaving the whole process behind, and I was able to reconnect with my life in an entirely natural way, forgetting the year I'd gone through. The holiday and the diving marked the end of my treatment. For me, diving meant taking up once again those things that I had to give up during that time. Therefore I was closing a chapter. Or so I thought. Returning home in September to start from where I'd left off a year ago, I noticed that my right arm was more swollen than the left one. I had heard of lymphedema, but according to doctors, it only affected some 10% of women, usually the elderly and people with low activity levels. So why was I getting it?

Lymphedema

At first I thought that by immobilizing my arm the swelling would subside. I thought it was temporary, the result of the effort made during the dives. I didn't know where to turn. Of all my doctors, none had left a phone number in case I should note symptoms like these, and my next appointment wasn't for more than a month.

I felt lost. I started looking for information on the Internet, and consulted a few people. I also started lymphatic drainage treatment, hoping that in five sessions my arm would be back to normal.

Two months later my arm was the same, but I had finally managed to locate a team of lymphedema specialists in Barcelona. I was able to understand a little better what this after-effect was. I also came to understand the huge lack of knowledge about it, and the scarcity of information and follow-up offered by the hospital. Once they have 'saved your life', the doctors fail to address the state you've been left in. They worry about a possible relapse of the tumour, but not about the after-effects because, at the end of the day, they've saved you from certain death – so why are you complaining?

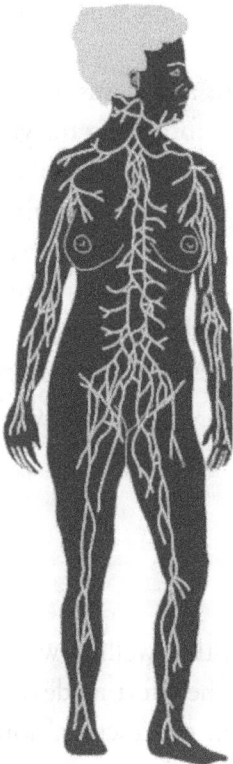

Lymphedema is the swelling of the body's soft tissues due to the accumulation of lymphatic fluid, usually in the limbs. It is the result of a malfunction of the lymphatic system, triggered either by genetic causes (primary lymphedema) or external causes such as the removal of lymph nodes (secondary lymphedema).

The lymphatic system is a circuit composed of vessels and nodes that, like the cardiovascular system, reaches every part of our body. Unlike the cardiovascular system, which flows in two directions – the arteries take blood away from the heart while the veins carry blood toward it – the lymphatic system is unidirectional. In other words, its only task is to collect lymph.

The arteries transport blood with nutrients and oxygen throughout the body. Part of the waste generated in this exchange is reabsorbed into the blood that continues its route towards the veins. But there is another part, comprising proteins, fats, etc. that the body eliminates through the lymphatic system. Consequently, the lymphatic system 'collects' this waste by making use of lymph, or lymphatic fluid.

While the blood has the heart to pump it around, the lymphatic system does not have a specific organ to pump its fluid. It primarily relies on the muscular and circulatory movement generated by the movement of the limbs. Unlike venous channels, lymphatic vessels are thinner, and the movement of fluids is rather slow and subtle.

The lymph reaches the lymph nodes, which are located at strategic points of the body (chest, armpits, groin, and neck). Their function is to filter the lymph and help the body recognize and fight germs and infections.

As we discussed in Chapter 4, in conventional treatments for breast surgery, whether mastectomy (total breast removal) or lumpectomy (tumour removal), surgeons generally remove at least the sentinel node for analysis.

They often remove the entire axillary node cluster to ensure that there are no tumour cells in the body. In doing so, they remove the natural lymph drainage pathway from the arm to the neck, in the arm located on the same side of the body that is operated on. Fortunately, this is not the sole return path for the fluid, so not everyone develops lymphedema.

However, the removal of these lymph nodes limits drainage and disrupts the normal balance of the entire body, sometimes needlessly. This is how lymphedema developed.

I could not believe it when it happened to me. I was making such a good recovery, and was so keen on putting the year of treatment behind me, and then I'm told this after-effect will be for life! I refused to accept it and I felt devastated.

I think it was the hardest time I'd experienced thus far. Having a swollen arm that you will have to take care of for the rest of your life, is, in itself, a drag.

But it meant more than this to me. For me, the lymphedema meant not being able to control everything, having 'failed' in my healing and recovery plans. It was completely unexpected. Mentally, I had intended to stay strong and positive until the end of treatment, because then it would be over. That was my goal. When the lymphedema appeared, my ability to take more blows and surmount more hurdles had come to an end. Suddenly, I was angry, raging at life, upset with both my doctors and myself.

Time and again I went over that conversation with the doctor who removed my lymph nodes 'per protocol', without listening to me. It seemed so terribly unjustifiable... It was the first time in my life I was faced with a predicament like this.

The consequences of that doctor's action was so serious that I could not move on or bypass it; a predicament that was the result having ignored my wish. I was infuriated. The swollen arm was there, and it would still be there because, according to the experts, it was permanent, nothing could change it. Moreover, it would gradually worsen.

The fury lasted a long time and, to this day, sometimes I lash out. Faced with the tumour, I never once pondered "why me?". I found scores of reasons. Not this time. I felt so powerless, so incensed! I couldn't get my head around it.

I frantically began to search for solutions. I went from total ignorance about lymphedema to immersing myself in a circuit that included lectures, courses, conferences, specialized centres and types of therapies. Before developing lymphedema myself, I felt fully informed on the subject, simply because I knew of its existence. Now I was to realize that I had much to learn.

I started having weekly lymphatic drainage sessions and doing specific exercises. I scoured the Internet to learn as much as I could about the different techniques used to treat lymphedema, including Nordic walking,[16] which they say encourages drainage in the arms and

---

16. Nordic walking is a recent sport invented by a Finnish cross-country skiing team in the 1930s in order to train in the summer. It involves walking at a brisk pace, holding poles similar to those used in skiing. When walking, the arms swing to

legs. I also began to go swimming two or three times a week. I did everything in my power, used everything available to me, to rid myself of the lymphedema.

Given that the swelling in my arm didn't go down as much as I would have liked, I went one step further. I found out about a new type of operation pioneered in Japan, which was being performed in Spain, specifically in Barcelona. So I jumped at the opportunity. Just to make this silly arm return to its normal size.

Now I clearly see how wrong I was, seeking solutions outside myself, treating my right arm with contempt instead of devoting special affection to it. I had a long way to go until I would understand this.

Supermicrosurgery for Lymphedema

I phoned the prestigious private clinic where this operation was being performed and had a preliminary interview with the doctor in charge of the process. He explained what the surgery involved: small superficial cuts are made in the forearm to access the lymphatic vessels just below the skin. By means of supermicrosurgery, these vessels are connected directly to the venous system, in order to drain lymph into the blood stream. Hence, by creating a new route by which to remove lymphatic fluid, the accumulation and stagnation problems are resolved. This reconnection process is called 'lymphaticovenous anastomosis'.

There is another possible technique, consisting in an autologous lymph node transplant. The nodes are usually extracted from the groin area and reimplanted in the armpit to replace the ones that have been removed. This second option aims to enable the lymphatic system to once again reabsorb the lymph produced by our limb.

---

the rhythm of the legs, in the opposite direction (when the right leg moves forwards, the right arm holds back). These movements improve blood circulation and drainage because they activate many muscles using a gentle pace.

I had several tests and went back to see the doctor. He had good news: my lymphedema was of the type that can be reabsorbed 100% because my lymph vessels were still working well, but I had to act quickly. And yet, although my initial prognosis was very good, they could not guarantee a reduction in volume of more than 30 to 60% of the lymphedema.

The operation, which takes some twelve hours, involves a week's stay in hospital, and a one-year rehabilitation process, with a compression bandage, swimming and a lymphatic drainage, depending on the doctor's prescription.

After providing me with all the relevant information, they drew up an estimate which far exceeded the price of a (very) high-end car. I left the clinic after the second appointment with a date for the operation, feeling over the moon. I did some numbers and then more numbers thinking how to get the money, because after all, what's more important than one's health? What better way to 'invest' our savings? I was already looking ahead to drawing a line under the whole process that had accompanied the tumour.

It was then, a few days later, when everything changed and I finally understood. I spoke to several friends and told them about my decision to undergo surgery again. I conveyed to them my state of mind, my desperation at seeing that my body would not let me move on as I always had done. And then, suddenly, I saw it clearly. It's amazing how the fog lifts, and everything that hitherto was fuzzy becomes clear. I suppose I was stumbling in the dark in search of solutions. Until I realized that my mistake lay precisely in believing, once again, that the solution to my problem was external to me. I could have the surgery, of course, I could yet again rush into an easy solution, take the plunge without fear, as I always had. But by doing so I was postponing the inner work I had to do. That of facing up to my fears and believing in myself, in my intuitions and my strength. I had spent my entire chemotherapy and radiotherapy treatments rejecting traditional methods, urging myself and others to take charge of their lives, with a view to taking responsibility for my health and my career. But, in fact, when the time came to make decisions, I didn't dare do anything radical. I thought (and still think) that chemo was not the right way to treat my tumour, but I did it. I thought (and still think) that it wasn't necessary to remove my lymph nodes, but in the end they did. I thought (and still think) that cancer is a process and that we are able to reverse it with our power, this and much more. But despite some minor changes in my life, I hadn't practised what I preached. At last, the time had come to face up to the truth. If I didn't do it now, my life would revert to a similar situation, until I was able to learn what I had to learn.

So I cancelled the operation. I had reached the point where I had to put into practice everything I so vehemently defended. And take a risk. To see life from the other side. I didn't change my mind in view of the operation's possible side effects: twelve hours anesthetized, a year of rehabilitation, that might or might not work, or even potentially bring about who-knows-what after-effects that today we still don't know about (probably nothing serious, but the procedure was in its infancy and the long-term results are unknown). I did it because a voice inside me urged me to take charge, to believe in myself and my resources, and prove it to myself.

The voice was strong and made me strong. I began to address the lymphedema with a very different approach. My right arm was no fool; on the contrary, it was a delicate arm and required more care and attention. My body wasn't a mess; on the contrary, it had summoned up all its strength during the entire chemotherapy process and had come out intact. My body had surmounted many other things over my thirty-seven years for which I had not even expressed my gratitude, dwelling only on what I didn't like about it (a kilo too much here, a wrinkle there, a big nose, sensitive skin), instead of thanking its strength, sensitivity, ability to regenerate, to adapt, and to improve itself. I suddenly remembered all those days, while I was walking the Way of Saint James, that I'd go to bed at night exhausted, my legs aching, and awakening the next day refreshed. I recalled that at that time I'd marvelled at the body's ability to recover from intense effort. I also remembered those late nights out in my youth. Whole weekends staying up all night, eating and drinking in excess. Different kinds of 'torture' to which I have submitted my body, such as long exposures to the sun, and those university examination periods. And my body never failed me.

I was determined to give myself another chance and let my body find its balance by helping it insofar as I could, accompanying it in its effort. Without aggressive techniques or operations but activities that would favour its equilibrium, stimulating drainage, and the circulation of energy.

I began to implement my new dynamic. Every day I would practise *qi gong* to recharge my energy pathways, to help my body to restore itself, to revitalize the lymph vessels. I no longer exercised as a short-term commitment, but as a routine. Swimming became part of my weekly activities. During my mountain hikes I got used to carrying two poles instead of one, to do Nordic walking. I continued with the lymphatic drainage once a week and I stopped carrying loads with the right arm. When cooking, I always wore a glove to protect it from cuts and splashes of oil, and was careful to avoid injury.

And I started to write this short book. Because **what I want most in this world is to share this experience with people who have experienced similar situations and do not find their inner strength**. I got tired of listening to others. There are too many voices, too many opinions and there is too much advice, and they are all external. When we pay attention to others we forget about ourselves.

I wanted, and I want each and every one of you, with or without a tumour, to be able to decide for yourselves, to find your own voice, and trust in your own judgement. Many self-help books speak in these terms, and often are useful. A year ago, I went to a book presentation that addressed precisely these issues. I asked the author how to move forward, with so much of our path in life still before us; in whom to believe. She told me the time of gurus, preachers and spiritual leaders was over. Now was the time to listen to ourselves and find our own answers and our way of being true to who we are. At the time, I don't think I took in the essence of her words as I do now. And that's how I intend to convey it and pass the baton to you.

Regarding my lymphedema, the obvious question hanging in the air is: what is the material outcome of this? To date the swelling has gone down by 60%. The 4 cm difference I had in the most swollen parts of my arm[17] is barely more than 2 cm. Its consistency has changed (the arm was hard, suggesting fibrosis in the tissue and meaning the fluid would be difficult to eliminate), and it's now soft and easy to squeeze.

Thus far I have had no infection or problem, and the only noticeable difference between it and my left arm is the compression sleeve that I wear every day.

Of course, sometimes it feels weaker and I don't believe this arm will ever be as it once was, it will never find its balance, or open up enough drainage channels. We are all human and fall into despair. If nothing else, I've learned to accept those moments as mine too, and live them rather than deny or hide them. It was thanks to this low moment, and the conversations resulting from it, that I decided not to have surgery, and instead recount my story. Just for that, everything has already made sense and has been worth it.

Chemo brain

There is ever more debate about this side effect. You can find out about it on the Internet. Hospitals are still not addressing it, or at least not in the same way they do concerning hair loss. Chemo brain refers to alterations in our powers of concentration, our memory, our attention span... both during chemotherapy and afterwards.

---

17. Lymphedema size is assessed by comparing the measurements of the circumference of both arms in six different points (hand, wrist, forearm, lower elbow, a point of the elbow, a point near the armpit). The six points of measurement do not change, and lymphedema monitoring consists of assessing the progression and trends of these perimeters.

After a session of chemotherapy, many patients have noted a sensation of being drugged or drunk. Obviously, we directly attribute this to the drugs, trusting that as they're eliminated from the body the symptoms will gradually disappear, as is the case of getting drunk and the subsequent hangover. The problem is that this is not always the case.

It's sometimes experienced as a kind of haze that prevents you from accessing your own memories. You feel muddled. Anecdotes or situations that you previously remembered clearly become fuzzy. You may not remember how you used to make an everyday cookery recipe, the ingredients you used, which of them you put in first or second. You may forget people's names, even those of friends or people in the neighbourhood. When trying to recall them, you know they're stored somewhere in your memory but have no access to them. You leave home and don't remember if you've turned off the light. You can't find your keys. The envelope that you'd put in your bag to post that morning isn't there when you get to the post-box, and you come home to find it on the table, because just before you left you took it out for no apparent reason. You read a book and get lost in what you read. It requires a huge effort to retain information. A friend tells you about her problems and after some time you've forgotten them. At a meeting, actions to be undertaken are assigned, and although you write them down they make no sense when you read over them. It's a challenge to organize yourself and set priorities. It also demands more effort to make decisions. And your movements may also become much clumsier.

This is most evident when you're tired, when you haven't slept. Even so, many experts cast doubt on the connection between chemotherapy and the problems described; basically, because we still haven't not found any quantifiable scientific evidence or direct relationship obtained through testing. Sometimes the cancer itself is attributed to these side effects. This is absurd because, in the case of my tumour, before treatment I was on the ball and as fit as a fiddle (I find it hard to believe that at the age of thirty-six I could suddenly lose some faculties and then recover them at thirty-eight). Or the blame is laid on a drop in the body's defences or malnutrition (my tests showed an impeccable physical recovery, yet the lapses continued). When you experience it for yourself, the symptoms become so evident and the relationship with chemo is so obvious that you don't need any study or additional corroboration. It's enough to spend time with the patient who suffers it and share their frustration.

It seems that cognitive problems arise because our nervous system and nerve cells are affected by treatment. Some schools of thought blame hormones for this change. Personally, I'm more convinced by the premise that associates chemo brain to medication. Not everyone gets the symptoms, although it is estimated that 70% of patients perceive it during treatment.

During my first cycle of chemotherapy, as they injected me with the drugs, I noticed changes in my body. I was reading the newspaper but was unable to continue, the letters seemed to dance before me. This reaction became more pronounced with each new cycle.

I was aware that it would be reckless to drive on the first day of each cycle. My reflexes were not as sharp as usual. But only upon recovery do you fully grasp how your faculties have been diminished, because the decline is progressive and you get used to it.

I experienced all the side effects I have described. My oncologist at the time attributed them to a drop in my defences, writing them off as trivial. I obviously would have preferred to have been warned beforehand about a series of side effects known as chemo brain.

When I finished the chemotherapy cycles, I thought I would be back to normal in three weeks. But the effects lasted much longer than I would have wished. By the time my hair had grown back, my blood tests were normal, I'd regained my skin tone and the fatigue was gone, I still had many cognitive lapses. During the chemo I continued doing some work, I read, did many puzzles and remained active. But when I wanted to get back into my work routine and regular activities the change and loss of my faculties became more apparent to me. I'd greatly simplified my life during treatment, and the whole experience was new, so I had nothing with which to compare it. But after a year, wanting to resume life and the work pace I was used to, I realized that everything I did called for extra effort and I wasn't performing at the level I was accustomed to.

First I took it philosophically, then I became angry, and then I decided to take charge of the matter without fear. I also decided to give myself time. So I made enquires, discovered what I am explaining here, and tried to put some little tricks into practice in my daily life to prevent oversights while I was recovering.

I read, and read copiously, and I still do puzzles, and work as before. At meetings I now take more notes to make sure I don't forget anything important, because sometimes even today I notice a fog in my brain that prevents me from accessing some memories. It's temporary, and I notice it more when I'm tired. I work harder to find the right words, or visualize the person with whom I had a certain conversation.

Some patients report that their effects are lasting for many years. For others they disappear after one or two years. As always, each person is different. And as I have often reiterated, patients have the right to be informed and also to know about this side effect, to give it the importance it has. Because when we know about it, we can help to prevent it and lessen its severity – through reading, physical exercise, food, everything we have at hand.

Infertility

One of the most troubling side effects can be infertility. I've heard so many different statistics related to the probability of chemotherapy damaging the reproductive system that I'd rather not stand by any in particular.

Clearly the risk exists. On the one hand, chemotherapy usually entails a common side effect: loss of menstruation or amenorrhea. It can happen at the start of treatment or after several cycles. Your period may return shortly after the last session, or it may take months. Regarding the consequences and side effects that we have discussed, each person reacts differently.

Sometimes menstruation does not return. Thus we enter the stage of menopause, often with its characteristic symptoms, such as hot flushes, which might have occurred even during treatment. When the patient is around fifty, this side effect is not usually much of a problem, but at thirty-five it may be entirely undesirable.

Don't forget, on the other hand, that the return of your period does not necessarily mean you will recover your fertility. The extremely aggressive nature of chemotherapy may often leave the reproductive system irreversibly damaged, leaving the egg cells or ovaries incapable of reproduction.

In Chapter 3 we discussed the options that exist today to safely and healthily preserve our ovarian tissue while we undergo chemotherapy. This tissue can be reimplanted a few years later, in the hope of producing eggs capable of being fertile. It is still not a widespread technique and, although optimistic, it cannot ensure a pregnancy.

The best we can do on our end is to try to minimize the impact of the chemotherapy on our reproductive system, both during and after treatment. I've said it here before: eat healthily, do exercise and use alternative therapies that stimulate the cleansing of the body and keep it in balance. Two good choices would be TCM plus either homeopathy or homotoxicology.

Less abundant hair

During treatment we dream of the moment when we can finally remove the wig and regain our usual appearance. But sometimes we may have a surprise, because our hair doesn't always grow back entirely. After treatment, some people have found themselves with white hair, whereas before they had hardly had a grey hair on them. Others have witnessed how their straight hair has turned curly. Some find that in certain patches their hair grows finer and less dense; sometimes not even that – and we aren't prepared for this last possibility. Age is usually a major factor involved in this after-effect. Older people's hair has less strength to withstand the treatment and restore itself; hence much of it gets lost along the way.

Faced with a situation such as alopecia, the alternatives are few. We can use a wig permanently, create a new image for ourselves with less hair, or resort to hair grafts. In some cases we can also use extensions to recover the former mane.

Don't forget that hair grows all over our body, and all of it may be affected. I know of women who saw their bikini line had grown down the groin, making their pubic hair more extensive. Others have commented that the hair on their legs had become longer, stronger or darker than before. Similarly, we may find that both our eyebrows and eyelashes thin out. From makeup to hair removal, a number of aesthetic techniques can help us. Although the most difficult and most important task will be to accept that our appearance has changed.

Numbness in the limbs

After several cycles of chemotherapy, it's not infrequent to notice a tingling sensation in the fingers and toes. The feeling may gradually increase, and it resembles what we feel when a limb has 'gone to sleep'. This is a mild version of the loss of sensitivity that occurs when, due to surgery or to a wound, the nerve endings conveying information to the brain are severed or broken. When these pathways are cut due to the action of a scalpel, our sense of touch is affected.

Chemotherapy toxins accumulate in different parts of the body, including nerve endings. As a result, the sensations in one's hands and feet may vary, with tingling and numbness. When these sensations start, you might assume that as your body gradually eliminates the toxins your limbs will return to normal. But this is not so. The process is not always automatic. The body may need a long time to recover, and your loss of touch may be permanent.

The feeling may be accompanied by joint pain similar to rheumatism. This is not an entirely crippling pain. It's especially noticeable in the morning, when you move the muscles after hours of immobility. Writing these notes I just realized that it no longer happens to me. I finished chemotherapy a year and nine months ago. When I began writing this book, I still noticed it.

I have a two-fold approach to this situation. First, we must ensure we purge from our body any cumulative toxicities, as much and as soon as possible. Second, we should take this process in our stride and accept the new peculiarities. Doctors estimate that it may take at least two years for the body to eliminate all the drugs you have received. So why not allow ourselves at least three years to find our balance and snap back?

Chest wall and lung damage

When we undergo radiotherapy, the healthy areas of our body also suffer the effects of radiation. What makes this treatment different from others is that we may begin to experience its side effects years after the treatment.

One of the most common side effects is fibrosis of the entire area. The tissues lose their elasticity and become harder. We can see at a glance this effect in the breast, which is tougher. But it can also occur in our internal organs, in both the chest wall and lungs.

This loss of flexibility may lead to complications and cause rib fractures, or a dry cough due to lung disease, etc. We must take into account that, after a long exposure to radiation, the adjacent area will be weakened and therefore be more vulnerable, and as a result more sensitive to infections.

It's just as probable that one hardly notices major changes and barely recalls radiotherapy treatment. Even so, it's always advisable to take extra care of the breast by regularly moisturizing it and protecting it from the sun and other types of harmful effects.

Freckles and moles

We've discussed how our skin suffers during chemotherapy. It dries out, loses its shine, and becomes more sensitive to the sun and even the cold; in some cases it becomes red. The melanin in the skin often reacts, especially in people with darker skin. These people may note how they tan even when they protect their skin.

Aside from these effects that usually go away, freckles, moles and even spots may appear. Moles usually begin as red dots. Over time, some acquire a characteristic dark brown tone. And these moles don't go away. Moreover, they may continue to appear once treatment has ended.

People with freckles will also see how these tiny blemishes multiply or intensify. Larger blotches, though not as common, can occur. The melanin in the skin reacts differently in each of us. The elderly are more prone to this effect, because with age the tendency for developing dark patches of skin is more natural.

Vein damage

The main reason why we are proposed to have a portacath implanted is to protect the veins from the direct aggression of the medication. Through the portacath the drug is dissolved directly into an abundant bloodstream which decreases the harm.

When chemotherapy is delivered into the arm veins, they become burnt. Their inner walls suffer and become inflamed. Initially, this reaction may cause pain or bruising, even at the precise moment the patient is receiving the medication. What starts as a normal reaction to an external aggression from the injected products can progress over time. The affected veins may collapse, harden and lose their flexibility. They may cease to function normally and small thrombi or clots may form inside them.

Usually this diagnosis is not serious. It can be successfully treated with special care at specific times and with guidelines on healthy behaviour. It's true that in many cases the vein will no longer be viable and will not be reused as a drug administration route or for blood draws.

Conclusions

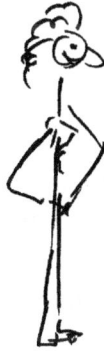

Throughout the pages of this book I've gradually shared with you what could be considered conclusions, guidelines or knowledge. Of course each woman, after her own experience, will have reached her own.

The following points reflect what, for me, have been the most important.

Move on

The past is the past. Just as the tumour process has a beginning it has an end. A new chapter in our life opens the day the tumour is discovered. Thus it's necessary to close the chapter in order to move on to the next. It's important to assimilate the experience into our life, yet it's equally important to let it fade with time and become a distant memory, jumbled up with new life experiences. We are not women with cancer, but women who have gone through a difficult situation at a given time. And that's all.

Our mind is very powerful

Learn to channel your strength and harness it to usher in positive thoughts, leaving no room for fear of what might happen.

This positive energy will always be to our advantage, in all areas of life, not only in sickness, and it will help us to better enjoy and be happier. To simply ensure this on a daily basis is already a great stride.

Live without feeling guilty

Little by little we can lighten the heavy load of obligations that we bear and not feel guilty about it. We all deserve a happy life without impositions or unsought sacrifices. We have every right to enjoy the little and big things that life has to offer without having to justify ourselves. We need nothing else. It's all about not setting yourself too high a standard, not analyzing yourself all the time, not judging yourself and not judging others.

We cannot control life

Things are what they are, not what we wish them to be. As much as we try to force them, life will always be stronger. If you fight to get what you want out of life and you don't, you can easily fall into frustration. However, if accept things as they are, adapt to what life has to offer, you will have fewer expectations, and each moment will be an unexpected gift. Until now, one of my fears was to miss out on the opportunities that life has to offer me. I finally realized that time, as its transpires, will provide us with endless opportunities, just as a river never stops letting water flow. Opportunity is not a train that stops only once at our station. It is a constant stream that allows us to choose between one and another option at our convenience.

We have the right to decide

The process that we have had to endure as a result of the emergence of a tumour need not be a standard experience or protocol in which we assent to what is imposed from outside. We have every right to know what is happening to us and to make decisions, regardless of the protocols. We are not numbers or statistics. We are people. Healing often rests upon how we feel, rather than the external treatment we may be administered. So it is important to feel comfortable with what we are doing.

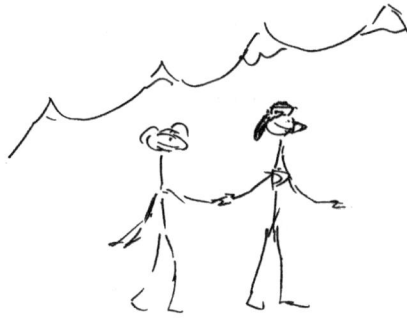

Take responsibility for our lives

Just as we have the right to decide how we want to tackle a tumour, taking responsibility involves proving ourselves as capable human decision-makers regarding our own lives. Just as we have the right to decide because we are responsible for any consequences, we are also responsible for ourselves and our health. To this end, we must be proactive and not just delegate our health issues to the doctor who is treating us. Our day-to-day outlook and the choices we make will shape us. The only ones responsible for the results we obtain will be ourselves. It all boils down to what we think, what we want, how we choose to nourish, take care of and pamper ourselves. So act boldly and take the initiative, make decisions that can help to improve your life: a change in habits, diet, a new alternative therapy that appeals to you – don't decide not to do it out of lethargy or to avoid raised eyebrows. It's irrelevant what people around us may think.

Convey our dissatisfaction

Doctors and nurses can get it wrong. Even though it may be the result of a decision with our best interest at heart, it still has a strong impact. If so, if your doctor has not done what you expected, or has been negligent, don't keep it inside: tell him or her. Be diplomatic and firm, but do it, act. It will be better for you, because you will have got it out of your system, and it will also be beneficial for him or her. It's important for professionals to become directly aware of the impact of their decisions.

Trust

Once we have overcome the hardship that goes hand in hand with treatment of the tumour, it's time to relax and trust in yourself and in life. We have done what we thought was most appropriate, at every step of the way, using everything at our disposal to recover. There is no room for regret or doubt. Now is not the time to think we could have done a little more, gone one step further. That stage is over, and now we begin a new one, that of serenity.

Associations and support groups

If you need help of any kind, either because you have lymphedema, or because you feel lonely, sad or different, remember that in most cities there are associations that provide support. More and more people are recovering from tumour treatments with every passing day and it's always a pleasure to know that your experience may be of help to someone else.

Reaching cruising speed

Looking ahead, a good way to approach life henceforth is to incorporate all these guidelines we have addressed in the conclusions, and that will help us lead a healthier life without major effort. Simple behaviour like thinking positively, caring about our diet, staying active, visiting an acupuncturist from time to time and having a reference book on our bedside table that will help us remember how we want to live our lives. These are the tricks that allow us to enjoy life and stop feeling guilty for everything that we do.

Bibliography
and other reference sources

General information about breast cancer

- **International Breast Cancer Awareness and Funding:** www.pinkribbon.org
- **National Cancer institute:** www.cancer.gov
- www.breastcancer.org
- **American Cancer Society:** www.cancer.org/
- **Wikipedia:** www.wikipedia.org
- **Anticancer:** A new way of life. Servan-Schreiber, David

Doctor Hamer

- **About Doctor Hamer:** http://dr-rykegeerdhamer.com/
- **The German/Germanic New Medicine:** www.newmedicine.ca

Tumour types and phases

Overview:
- **American Cancer Society:** www.cancer.org/cancer/breastcancer/overviewguide/breast-cancer-overview-what-is-breast-cancer
- **National Cancer Institute:** www.cancer.gov/cancertopics/types/breast

Location:

- www.cancer.org/cancer/breastcancer/overviewguide/breast-cancer-overview-what-is-breast-cancer

Biology:

- **WebMD:** www.webmd.com/breast-cancer/breast-cancer-types-er-positive-her2-positive

Stage:

- **American Cancer Society:** www.cancer.org/cancer/breastcancer/detailedguide/breast-cancer-staging

Grade:

- **National Cancer Institute:** www.cancer.gov/cancertopics/factsheet/detection/tumor-grade

Traditional Chinese Medicine

- **Traditional Chinese Medicine World (TCMWF) Foundation:** www.tcmworld.org
- **TCM and Breast Cancer:** www.breastcancer.com.

Artificial fertilization techniques

- **Cryopreservation of ovarian tissue.** Basic concepts.
- **MyOncofertility.org.** http://myoncofertility.org/animations/ovarian_tissue_cryopreservation_basics
- **Natural Cycle IVF.** www.naturalcycleivf.com/

Patients' rights

- **Simon P. "Diez mitos en torno al consentimiento informado".** Revista Anales. (Only Spanish)

- **WMA Declaration of Lisbon on the Rights of the Patient.** www.wma.net/en/30publications/10policies/l4/

Nutrition

- **Journal of Inflammation:** www.journal-inflammation.com.
- **National Center for Biotechnology Information (NCBI):** www.ncbi.nlm.nih.gov/.
- **European Food Information Council (EFIC):** www.eufic.org/.
- **US National Library of Medicine:** www.ncbi.nlm.nih.gov/pubmed

Some articles:
- **Nutrition and Survival After the Diagnosis of Breast cancer:** A Review of the evidence. Demark-Wahnerfried. J Clin Oncol 20: 3302-3316. 2002.
- **Can Lifestyle Modification Increase Survival in Women Diagnosed with Breast cancer.** Cheryl L. Rock. J. Nutr. 132: 3504S-3509S, 2002.

Lymphedema

- **The Lymphoedema support network (UK):** www.lymphoedema.org/
- **The National Lymphedema Network:** www.lymphnet.org/home.htm
- **Supermicrosurgery for Lymphoedema:** www.ouh.nhs.uk/services/departments/lymphoedema/default.aspx

Bibliography

EMOTO, Masaru. *The Hidden Messages in Water.* Atria Books

FISZBEIN, Varda. *Agua y conciencia.* Ediciones Obelisco

LAVIER, Jacques-André. *Médecine chinoise, médecine totale.* Grasset

MAMBRETTI, Giorgio y SERAPHIN, Jean. *Medicine Upside Down: What If Hamer Was Right?* Blossoming Books

MORITZ, Andreas. *Cancer Is Not A Disease - It's A Survival Mechanism.* Ener-Chi.com

—. *Timeless Secrets of Health and Rejuvenation.* Ener-Chi.com

—. *Lifting the Veil of Duality.* Ener-Chi.com

SERVAN-SCHREIBER, David. *Anticancer: A new way of life.* Michael Joseph

SCHWARZ, Mario. *Medicina tradicional china.* Deva's

SILVERMAN, Dan y DAVIDSON, Idelle. *Your Brain After Chemo.* DaCapo Press

YOUNG, Robert y Shelley. *The Ph Miracle: Balance Your Diet, Reclaim Your Health.* Grand Central Publishing.

ANNEXES

DECALOGUE OF THE PATIENTS. DECLARATION OF BARCELONA OF PATIENTS' ASSOCIATIONS 2003.

On May 20 and May 21, 2003, Barcelona played host to a meeting attended by health professionals and representatives from patient organizations and associations and health service from across Spain. The purpose of the meeting was to obtain information on the views and experiences of patients and their constituencies in six areas of interest on which work had been prepared prior to the event. The organization and presentation of the information obtained is known as the Barcelona Declaration of Patients' Associations, which is summarized as the Patients' Decalogue[18].

1. Contrasted quality information respecting the plurality of the sources

Patients need information of contrasting quality according to explicit accreditation criteria and provided by professionals, preferably doctors. Respect for the many diverse sources and information agents

---

18. Source AECC, the Spanish Association Against Cancer (www.aecc.es). Statements: www.aecc.es/SobreElCancer/bibliotecadedocumentos/Documents/%20 nacionales/decálogo%20of%20the%20pacientes.pdf.

must be contemplated. Information must be produced in a comprehensible language and adapted to the understanding capacity of the patients.

2. Decisions focused on the patient

Decisions regarding medical treatment must be guided by medical judgement based on the best scientific knowledge available but heeding, whenever possible, the patient's will and his/her explicit preferences with regards to quality of life and the results expected from such treatment.

3. Respect for the values and autonomy of the informed patient

When health decisions lead to different alternatives according to the values and preferences of each specific patient, the commitment of a democratic society with respect for the dignity and autonomy of its members recommends advances in the development of measures to facilitate maximum adjustments between the options chosen and desired by correctly informed patients.

4. Relationship doctor-patient based on the mutual respect and trust

The importance of a doctor-patient relationship is defined as a fundamental relationship based on respect and mutual trust that leads to the improvement and/or resolution of the health problems and quality of life of patients and their relatives. Associations may help improve this relationship and help it to develop in a more symmetrical way.

5. Specific education and training on communication skills for professionals

Health systems must create specific training opportunities in communication skills for their professionals and within organizations so that a more symmetrical and satisfactory doctor-patient communication relationship may be possible for patients.

6. Participation of the patients in the determination of priorities in the health care

All citizens, especially patients, and the organizations that represent them have to take a more active role in determining priorities that define their access to health services and help identify value and satisfy their health needs.

7. Formal democratization of the sanitary decisions

In a health system focused on patients, the existence of formal mechanisms that favour greater participation of citizens in the defining of public policies related to health care must be promoted through the application of existing laws.

8. Recognition of the patients' organizations as agents of the health policy

Patient associations and organizations that represent them play a fundamental role in helping to introduce approved laws and promoting better communication between scientific societies, Health Administrations and individual patients.

9. Improvement of the patients' knowledge of their basic rights

The patient must have more information and knowledge regarding his/her rights, which must be provided by health professionals. This is one of their basic rights.

10. Guarantee of fulfilment of the patients' basic rights

Correct implementation of the patients' rights and evaluation of their compliance within the evaluation strategies of health quality must be guaranteed.

Annex 2

CLASSIFICATION OF FOODS

based on the body's pH

Type of food	Alcalinity			Acidity		
	+++	++	+	+	++	+++
Oils	Olive	Linsead		Sunflower		
Sweeteners	Stevia	Marple syrup, rice syrup	Unrefined honey and sugar	Processed honey	White sugar	Artificial sweeteners
Fruits	Lemon, watermelon, grapefruit, mango, papaya	Dates, figs, melon, grapes, papaya, kiwi, bilberry/blueberry, apple, pear, raisins	Orange, banana, cherry, pineapple, peach, avocado	Plum	Morello cherry, strawberry, pineapple	Blackberry, cranberry, prune
Vegetables	Asparagus, onions, parsley, raw spinach, broccoli, garlic	Pumpkin, green beans, beetroot, celery, lettuce, courgette/zucchini, sweet potato	Carrot, tomato, sweet corn/maize, mushrooms, cabbage, peas, artichoke, olive, soya bean, tofu	Cooked spinach, Brussels sprouts	Canned products, frozen products, mushrooms	Vegetables in brine
Seeds and dried fruits		Almonds	Chestnuts	Pumpkin and sunflower seeds	Peanut, walnut, chocolate	
Cereals			Wild rice, quinoa, millet, amaranth	Spelt, brown rice, oats, rye	Rice, corn/maize, buckwheat	Wheat, white flour, cakes, pastries
Dairy products			Goat milk, goat cheese	Butter, yogurt, cottage cheese	Sweetened yogurt	Cow cheese, cow milk
Meat and eggs				Eggs	Turkey, chicken, lamb	Veal, pork
Fish				Blue Fish		Seafood, canned fish
Condiments				Vinegar	Mayonnaise, ketchup, mustard, soya sauce	
Drinks	Infusions	Green tea		Black tea	Coffee, wine	Beer, non-alcoholic beverages

Annex 3

GLYCEMIX INDEX TABLE

The complete list of the glycemic index and glycemic load for more than 1,000 foods can be found in the article "International tables of glycemic index and glycemic load values: 2008" by Fiona S. Atkinson, Kaye Foster-Powell, and Jennie C. Brand-Miller in the December 2008 issue of **Diabetes Care**, Vol. 31, number 12, pages 2281-2283.[19]

---

19. http://care.diabetesjournals.org/content/31/12/2281.long

GLYCEMIX INDEX TABLE[20]

FOOD	Glycemic index (glucose = 100)
VEGETABLES	
Carrots	35
Green peas	51
Instant mashed potato	87
Parsnips	52
Sweet potato	70
Yam	54
BEANS AND NUTS	
Baked beans	40
Black beans	30
Blackeye peas	33
Cashews, salted	27
Chickpeas	10
Kidney beans	29
Lentils	29
Navy beans	31
Peanuts	7
Soy beans	15
GRAINS	
Brown rice	50
Bulgur	48
Couscous	65
Pearled barley	28
Quick cooking white basmati	67

20. This table is an extract of the summary published by the Harvard Health Publications. www.health.harvard.edu/newsweek/Glycemic_index_and_glycemic_load_for_100_foods.htm

FOOD	Glycemic index (glucose = 100)
GRAINS	
Quinoa	53
Sweet corn on the cob	60
White rice	89
FRUITS	
Apple	39
Banana	62
Dates	42
Grapefruit	25
Grapes	59
Orange	40
Peach	42
Pear	38
Prunes	29
Raisins	64
Watermelon	72
DAIRY PRODUCTS AND ALTERNATIVES	
Ice cream, premium	38
Ice cream, regular	57
Milk, full fat	41
Milk, skim	32
Reduced-fat yogurt with fruit	33
PASTA and NOODLES	
Fettucini	32
Macaroni	47
Spaghetti, white, boiled	46
Spaghetti, wholemeal	42
BREAKFAST CEREALS AND RELATED PRODUCTS	
All-Bran™	55
Cornflakes™	93

FOOD	Glycemic index (glucose = 100)
BREAKFAST CEREALS AND RELATED PRODUCTS	
Muesli	66
Oatmeal	55
Puffed wheat	80
Raisin Bran™	61
Special K™	69
BAKERY PRODUCTS AND BREADS	
100% Whole Grain™ bread	51
Baguette, white, plain	95
Corn tortilla	52
Hamburger bun	61
Kaiser roll	73
Pita bread, white	68
Pumpernickel bread	56
Wheat tortilla	30
White wheat flour bread	71
Whole wheat bread	71
COOKIES AND CRACKERS	
Graham crackers	74
Rice cakes	82
Rye crisps	64
Shortbread	64
Soda crackers	74
Vanilla wafers	77
BEVERAGES	
Apple juice, unsweetened	44
Orange juice, unsweetened	50
Tomato juice, canned	38
Coca Cola®	63
Fanta®, orange soft drink	68

FOOD	Glycemic index (glucose = 100)
SWEETENERS	
Fructose	19
Glucose	99
Honey	61
Sacarose	68

HOW TO WEAR A BUFF®

Instructions provided by BUFF®, which manufactures this multifunctional fabric headwear.

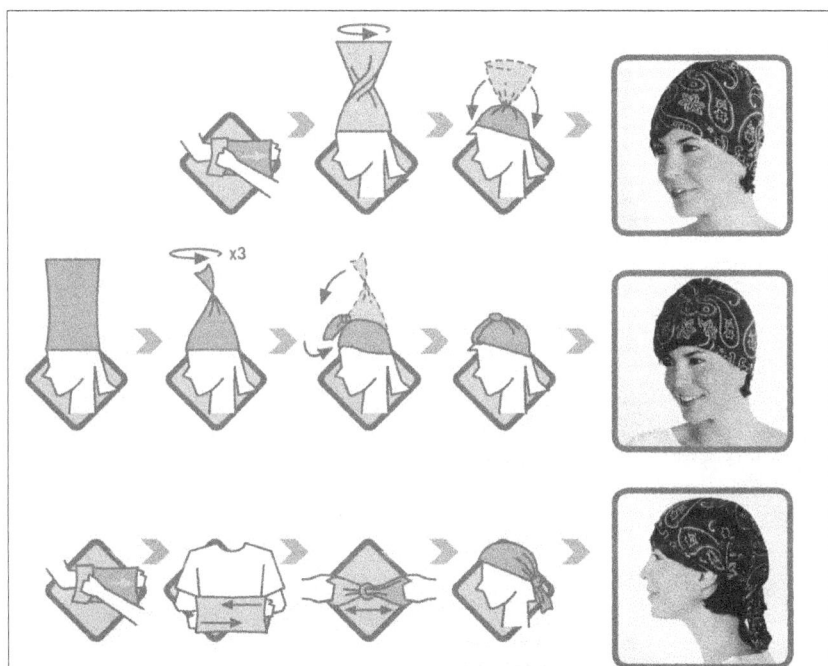

Annex 5

TIMELINES

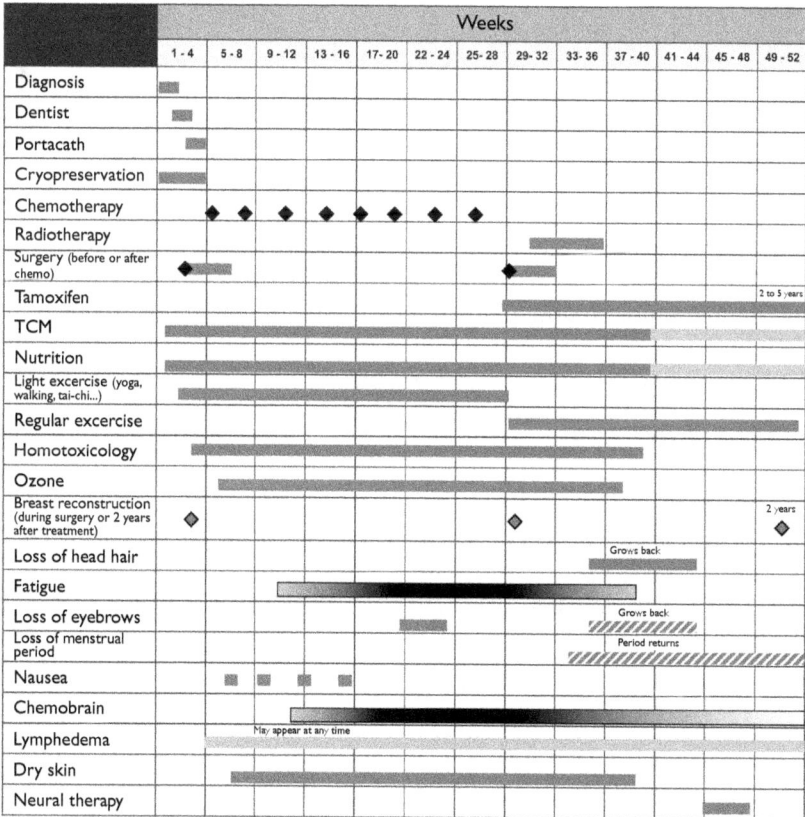

	Weeks												
	1 - 4	5 - 8	9 - 12	13 - 16	17- 20	22 - 24	25- 28	29- 32	33- 36	37 - 40	41 - 44	45 - 48	49 - 52
Diagnosis													
Dentist													
Portacath													
Cryopreservation													
Chemotherapy													
Radiotherapy													
Surgery (before or after chemo)													
Tamoxifen													2 to 5 years
TCM													
Nutrition													
Light excercise (yoga, walking, tai-chi...)													
Regular excercise													
Homotoxicology													
Ozone													
Breast reconstruction (during surgery or 2 years after treatment)													2 years
Loss of head hair									Grows back				
Fatigue													
Loss of eyebrows									Grows back				
Loss of menstrual period									Period returns				
Nausea													
Chemobrain													
Lymphedema		May appear at any time											
Dry skin													
Neural therapy													

About the author

Teresa Ferreiro (1972) studied Communication Sciences at the Universidad Complutense of Madrid. Subsequently she completed a training programme for Young Talents at the IMD Business School. As a communication expert, she has developed her professional career in various multinational companies and institutions based in a number of countries, heading a variety of business projects.

At present, Teresa continues her professional career in the fields of research, communication and project management. Her experience with breast cancer and the knowledge she garnered from it – the subject of this book – has also led her to collaborate as a speaker in debates, conferences and conventions to convey the messages she supports and build analogies around them.

Her genuine interest in people has urged her to take a path in search of meaning and openness, along which she continues to advance day by day. The author considers her breast tumour as just one of life's many experiences which may leave a deep mark on us but not necessarily become the turning point of our life.

*
**

Carlos Cordón is professor at IMD business school. His areas of interest are supply and demand chain management, strategic management and outsourcing. Other interests include leadership and project management. He is the author of numerous articles and case studies for which he has won various awards. Carlos Cordón is also the author of several books including "The Power of Two".